Dare...
to Make Love with 2, 3, 4... or More

What I love
Is to make love
With the 3 of us.
It's absolutely out.
I know it's hippie shit.
But I say it loud:
With the 3 of us... I love it.
What I love
Is to be caressed by four hands.
If one is tired, the next one is fit.
With the 3 of us... uh! I love it!

— from "Love with the 3 of Us,"
translation of original French lyrics written
by Françoise Cactus, lead singer of the
German-French pop group Stereo Total

Titles in the Dare... series

Dare... to Have Anal Sex by Coralie Trinh Thi

Dare... to Have Sex Everywhere but in Bed by Marc Dannam

Dare... to Try Bisexuality by Pierre Des Esseintes

Dare... to Try Bondage by Axterdam

Dare... to Try Kama Sutra by Marc Dannam and Axterdam

Vacation Sex Quiz Book by Marc Dannam and Axterdam

Ordering

Trade bookstores in the U.S. and Canada please contact:

Publishers Group West
1700 Fourth Street, Berkeley CA 94710
Phone: (800) 788-3123 Fax: (800) 351-5073

Hunter House books are available at bulk discounts for textbook course adoptions; to qualifying community, health-care, and government organizations; and for special promotions and fund-raising. For details please contact:

Special Sales Department
Hunter House Inc., PO Box 2914, Alameda CA 94501-0914
Phone: (510) 865-5282 Fax: (510) 865-4295
E-mail: ordering@hunterhouse.com

Individuals can order our books from most bookstores, by calling **(800) 266-5592**, or from our website at
www.hunterhouse.com

Marc Dannam

Dare...

to Make Love with 2, 3, 4... or More

Hunter House

Hunter House Inc., Publishers
PO Box 2914
Alameda CA 94501-0914

Library of Congress Cataloging-in-Publication Data

Dannam, Marc.
[Osez—faire l'amour à 2, 3, 4—]
Dare — to make love to 2, 3, 4—or more / Marc Dannam. — 1st ed.
p. cm. — (Dare... series)
Includes bibliographical references.
ISBN 978-0-89793-512-8
1. Sexual intercourse. 2. Triangles (Interpersonal relations) 3. Group sex. 4. Sex instruction. I. Title. II. Title: Dare to make love to two, three, four or more.

HQ31.D2237 2010
306.77—dc22 2010005844

Project Credits

Cover Design: Brian Dittmar Graphics
Cover Illustrator: Arthur de Pins
Book Production: John McKercher
Translator: Robert Nighthawk
Copy Editor: Amy Bauman
Managing Editor: Alexandra Mummery
Publishing Assistant: Martha Scarpati
Publicity Coordinator: Sean Harvey
Order Fulfillment: Washul Lakdhon
Administrator: Theresa Nelson
Computer Support: Peter Eichelberger
Senior Marketing Associate: Reina Santana
Rights Coordinator: Candace Groskreutz
Customer Service Manager: Christina Sverdrup
Publisher: Kiran S. Rana

Printed and bound by Bang Printing, Brainerd, Minnesota
Manufactured in the United States of America

9 8 7 6 5 4 3 2 1 First Edition 10 11 12 13 14

Contents

Note: Some books quoted in this work have English-language editions; our text is translated from the French original and may not match the exact wording of the published English text.

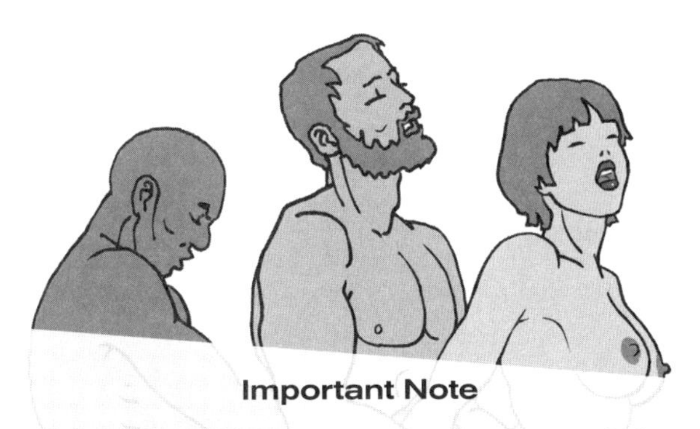

Important Note

The material in this book is intended to provide a review of information regarding the exploration of one's sexuality with multiple partners. Every effort has been made to provide accurate and dependable information. We believe that the sensuality advice given in this book poses no risk to any healthy person. However, if you have any sexually transmitted diseases, we recommend consulting your doctor before using this book.

Therefore, the publisher, authors, and editors, as well as the professionals quoted in the book, cannot be held responsible for any error, omission, professional disagreement, or dated material, and are not liable for any damage, injury, or other adverse outcome of applying any of the information resources in this book. If you have questions concerning the application of the information described in this book, consult a qualified professional.

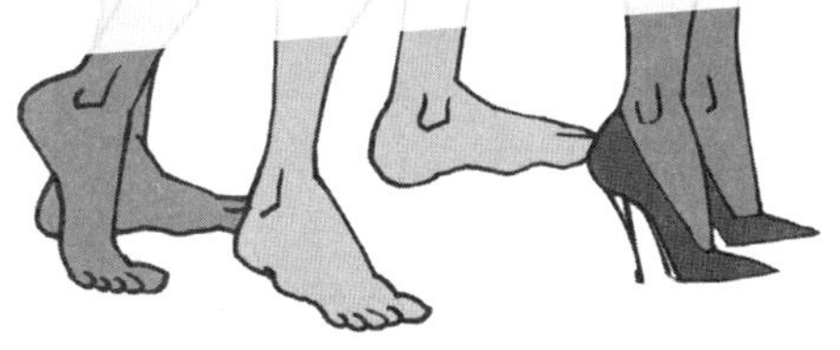

Foreword to the U.S. Edition

by Yvonne K. Fulbright, PhD

...the Series

Leave it to the superbly sensual French to make the exotic all the more erotic, enticing, and accessible with the most charming set of sex books ever released.

When I first saw the *Osez...* (Dare) series, I was instantly seduced by the playful, titillating covers of this set of more than twenty pocket books. Delightfully disarming, these works inspire one to take on all taboos, summoning lovers to unleash their sexual nature as never before. Talk about *ooh-là-là*—these books leave no doubt as to why the French are known the world over for being sexy. Whether it is their food, wine, fashion, or simply their sensual language, the French are credited with and revered for encouraging eroticism.

Throw the word *French* in front of any English word(s)—whether it is *French* underwear, *French* maid outfit, *French* kiss, or *French* champagne—and it is suddenly sexy. And this French book is no exception. Translated into Portuguese, Spanish, and Italian, it is now available in English for your delight. It charms countless lovers to "carpe diem" and urges them to seek their pleasure as never before.

...this Book

Warning: You may never look at sex the same way after reading this book. French writer Mark Dannam is about to take you on a frank and fearless "sexcapade" involving more fingers, skin, lips, and loins at the same time than you would have thought possible. And he doesn't hold back. All that is titillating and taboo is fair game in the following pages, with Dannam, author of sixteen other books from the original *Osez...* (Dare) series, touching on topics that few writers dare to explore—like swinging and gang bangs. Whether you plan to act on his advice or are simply looking to amplify your arousal, this book will not disappoint.

Sex with more than one person can be traced back through human history. The Canaanites, for example, are known to have indulged in elaborate orgies in an attempt to invite their rain god to water the crops for a bountiful harvest. With Dannam, however, things are already wet, and bound to get wetter, as he prepares and guides lovers to successfully navigate the pleasures that are to be had with more than one partner at the same time. Meant for lovers of all sexual orientations and offering any and all combinations of multiple-partner sex, this book includes resources and inspirations to invite even more action.

...a frank and fearless "sexcapade" involving more fingers, skin, lips, and loins at the same time than you would have thought possible...

It doesn't take a sexologist and sex educator like myself to tell you that having sex with more than one person isn't for everyone—and others may shame you for it. But whether you're looking to experiment, hoping to invite the occasional partner into your coupledom, or seeking to make *ménages-à-trois* or group-sex situations a regular occurrence, Dannam helps you do it and without judgment. From the rules for safer sex to seductions to positions for exploring each lover, Dannam does everything but get in on the action with you. He equips you with everything you need to know to realize your full potential for "coming" in new and forbidden ways. He dares you to do, say, and dream about things that most sex writers aren't even attuned to when it comes to "moresome" explorations. In this book, no one says, "Three's a crowd." Everyone's invited to the party. So be sure to *amusez-vous bien!*

— Yvonne K. Fulbright, PhD, MSEd
Professor of Human Sexuality, Argosy University
Author of *Touch Me There!* and *The Hot Guide to Safer Sex*;
coauthor of *Your Orgasmic Pregnancy*

Introduction

Going to bed with two lovers? Three lovers? Even more?! You've never thought about it? Of course you have.

So you've decided to take on multiple partners. No doubt this decision comes after carefully considering the idea and how it jives with your own principles, or—if you're jumping in as part of a couple—with your partner's principles as well. This guide aims to give you some practical advice—for example, ideas about positions and situations that you can try out—and to whet your appetite for adventure by offering some sexy stories about people who have gone down this road before you.

My focus won't be on those sexual encounters, often quick and impersonal, that take place in swingers clubs. Even if they're technically part of the subject, I want to focus on relationships that take place in more intimate settings, between partners who have a whole night in front of them and who are exploring their sexuality far away from prying eyes. Because of this, I am also not going to ramble on about the possibility or impossibility of living long-term in a *ménage à trois* (threesome).

Finally, I won't discuss theories about why polyamory is emerging in Western societies—a development that in some ways mimics the polygamy that Eastern societies have long practiced. Just remember this simple definition of polyamory:

> **"(from gr. *poly*: many and lat. *amor*: love). A new term introduced by certain advocates of multiple, simultaneous erotic relationships. According to their definition, polyamory is based on a conscious decision not to limit one's erotic potential and to engage in several or even many relationships at the same time as long as they are all based on honesty, integrity, and mutual caring. The very broad definition thus covers, among other things, not only monogamous 'open' marriages, but also group marriages and 'intimate networks.'"**
>
> — http://www2.hu-berlin.de/sexology/GESUND/ARCHIV/CDS.HTM#P

And remember, too, that polyamory is a recently coined word, dating from the 1960s.

But that's another story. What I'm focusing on here is sexual practices, and I have three audiences in mind. One audience is made up of those of you who have already had the pleasure of an extra guy or girl in your bed. For you, this book may bring back happy memories. It may call up a few regrets as well, but if so, it will hopefully help heal those wounds. This book is also for those of you who want to try multiple partners but have never dared to do so because you fear seeming silly, being clumsy, or looking baffled in what would be a novel situation. Finally, the third group I have in mind includes those of you who don't really want to try this out with anyone but simply want to read this book about those who do, as part of your exploration of the sociology, literature, and practice of eroticism.

ch 1. Preparation

Threesomes and swinging go back a long way. One can find an odd scene sculpted in relief on the *Portail de la Vierge* (Portal of the Virgin), the western doorway of Paris's Notre Dame Cathedral. At the base of the scene, which includes a likeness of Virgin Mary, three panels depict the story of Eve: her birth, her sin, and her punishment. But the circumstances under which she bites the apple are not those you learned in school. Instead of a serpent, a nude woman shooting up from the Tree of Knowledge represents temptation. Adam and Eve stand to her sides, their genitals covered with leaves, and Eve is shown biting into an apple. The nude woman, who has a serpent's tail, is Lilith, Adam's first wife, who had been banished from Eden by God because she was too lewd. So what are we to conclude from this relief? Maybe multiple partners were involved in the original sin and Lilith was planning on suggesting something sexual and illicit to the young couple, who certainly wouldn't have refused.

More recently, in the French book *Super positions*—a history of sex positions—authors Anna Alter and Perrine Cherchève describe some very early representations of multiple partners. As they note, "[P]rofessor Emmanuel Anati [a paleontologist] has, in his collection of reproductions of cave paintings, several scenes of sexual acts involving more than two people. In Mongolia, Nora Novgorodova, a Russian specialist in bone art, excavated representations of homosexual relations involving three people."

The ancient Greeks also depicted threesomes in their art. The vase below (see Figure 1.1), which was painted in 510 BC, shows a hetaera (a Greek courtesan) being taken doggy-style by a bearded man while she sucks off another man who is standing in front of her.

Another vase depicts three partners together: A naked woman is offering herself to a man while a second man, with an erection, holds her up.

Japanese prints from a later date demonstrate that similar practices went on all around the world. According to Alter and Cherchève, illustrations from a medical book written around

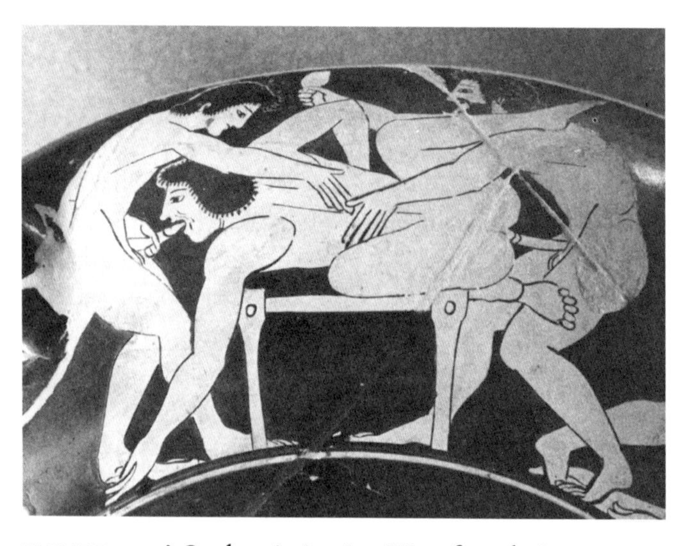

FIGURE 1.1. **A Greek antiquity circa 510 BC from the Louvre showing a threesome (from Wikimedia Commons, the free media repository © Marie-Lan Nguyen)**

710 CE show several threesomes going on at once. The authors note, "Here, a courtesan is in her client's bed. She slides under the covers to join her lips with those of her true love, who is also in bed with the client. Further away, the owner of a bordello initiates a young female lodger who is leaning on the arms of an experienced whore. In the background, a Japanese man joins a beautiful boy while, with his left hand, massaging his jealous wife's genitals."

High reliefs carved in the tenth century at the Temple of Lakshmana in Khajuraho, India, depict ritual orgies that involve many couples tangled together (see Figure 1.2). The temple walls offer many similar scenes.

In the centuries since, many more depictions of pleasure parties have appeared. A book by Nicolas Chorier from the

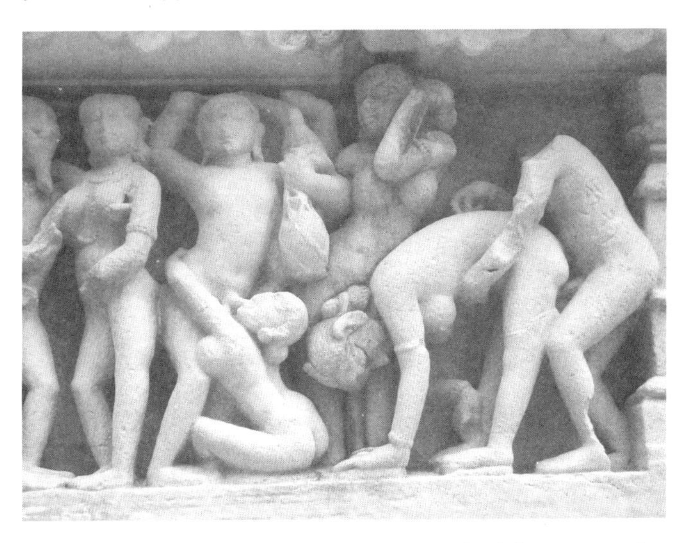

FIGURE 1.2. **An erotic detail from the base of Lakshmana Temple in Khajuraho, India (from Wikimedia Commons, the free media repository)**

seventeenth century entitled *School of Women* or *Dialogues of Luisa Sigea* features engravings showing several couples having sex in the same room. In the eighteenth century, things really explode: Literature and art abound with scenes of lovemaking between three, four, or more people, while police reports document real orgies.

Since then, of course, things haven't changed.

Mind you, it turns out that art isn't reflecting life so much as fantasy—many more people say they fantasize about multiple partners than actually engage in multiple partner sex. In July of 2000 a French marketing organization conducted a poll for the magazine *Marie Claire*, asking French men and women about their fantasies. Thirty-four percent of men reported fantasizing about making love to two women, while only 11 percent of women imagined having sex with multiple partners. When we look at real acts, though, we find substantially lower numbers are reported. A different study found that 10 percent of men and only 2 percent of women say that they've had sex with two people at the same time.

The numbers are much higher in certain groups, however. According to a third study by the marketing agency Ispos, business executives are the real enthusiasts of multiple partners—21 percent said they had tried it.

From such information, one might conclude that people engaging in sex with two or more partners are still a minority, and that this practice is rare enough that some sexologists and sociologists talk about it as if it played no role at all in people's lives. In the book *La Vie sexuelle en France* (Sexual Life in France), sociologist Janine Mossuz-Lavau writes, "I've met a few men and somewhat fewer women who have tried threesomes at some point in their lives." "A few" does not sound like many; "at some point in their lives" is not often.

Yet every weekend, hundreds of swingers clubs in France and the United States fill up with couples and even singles, as do the back rooms of gay nightclubs, and according to Jessica Bennett from *Newsweek*, "Researchers are just beginning to study the phenomenon, but the few who do estimate that openly polyamorous families in the United States number more than half a million." Meanwhile, Internet forums and magazines directed at swingers and other members of the polyamorous community print thousands of messages from people looking for multiple partners. Today there are even poly blogs, podcasts, and online magazines (most notably *Loving More*; www.lovemore.com) catering to this community. True, the small visibility of polyamory doesn't make it a mass movement and public attention is largely helped along by the media, which has discovered a source of eye-catching stories, but even if this type of sexual exploration is restricted to a minority, that still means thousands of people are giving themselves over to multiple partners every day. Why not you, too?

The Taboo So here's the norm: two people having sex. They can be heterosexual or homosexual; they may have been together for years, or they may be recently acquainted. Today, pretty much everything that can possibly happen between two consenting adults in bed (or, for that matter, on the floor of the living room) is an acceptable part of sexual life. Few activities—not fellatio, anal sex, spanking, S&M, or the use of sex toys—are seen as a transgression against the order of things, but put a third or fourth person in the bed, and that changes the story. This might seem strange to say when today's magazines freely talk about partner swapping and swingers show up on television, but it is true. You may notice that few of your friends will admit to having had multiple partners without a dose of (false?) modesty. Even more embarrassing is to confess to doing it often and enjoying it. Any man who admits to that will immediately be considered a pervert, a consenting woman will be tossed into the category of "slut," and both may quickly become objects of contempt and lecherous curiosity.

Thinking about multiple partners—that's both common and normal. But realize the fantasy is rare, and probably a day to remember for those involved. It means entering a situation loaded with voyeurism and exhibitionism. Someone, whether stranger or friend, will see you having sex. So will your regular partner if he or she is in on it. And if you've only been in heterosexual relationships until now, you, too, will have the opportunity to develop another side to your sexuality: contact with someone of the same sex. Even when playing heterosexual games with multiple partners, it would be odd if you didn't end up caressing partners of your same gender now and then. As you'll find out, that's part of the fun.

Having sex with two, three, or more partners will thus catapult you into a universe of new experiences. Even if the eternal methods of physical love remain the same—stroking, fellatio, cunnilingus, vaginal and anal penetration, etc.—they take on a new intensity when experienced with a third person.

◎ **Taking the Plunge** Why do we want it?

According to most psychologists, the desire to have a threesome is seen as an ancient fantasy that is often linked to the three component parts of the well-known Oedipus complex (the mother, the father, and the child). In the mind, it can have one of three points of origin: The unconscious development of this fantasy could be a result of voyeurism or exhibitionism, an unconscious means of living out a hidden homosexual/bisexual desire, or a way to discover whether one of the partners will allow the other to cheat.

One of the best reasons to invite a third person into bed once in a while is to indulge your fantasies, perhaps with the understanding that "what happens in your bed, stays in your bed." Although this decision requires careful thought and planning, it ultimately promises to be a lot of fun, as the comments of this Internet user, unfortunately anonymous, attest:

> **"I've had lots of experiences with a FFM [female–female–male] trio. They are never short, because the women like to make it heady: They like to get to know each other, appreciate each other, before, after, and during.... The trios that I've been in were very sapphic. Sometimes, the third girl was lesbian rather than bi.... The advantage of being in a threesome with two members of the same sex who are both bi is that there is no distance between them, and this offers its own possibilities. You can have fun for a long time...and get some pleasure...."**

Although more rare, there is another way of doing things that reverses the common function of threesomes, which is to allow one partner to explore his or her homosexuality. Some threesome situations allow two homosexual women to treat themselves to a hetero interaction every once in a while. At least, that's what this woman, posting on the same forum as the man above, says:

> **"I live with a woman (we're a lesbian couple). We have a three-way relationship with a male friend, and everything is going well. We're still at the beginning, but I can tell you that this is different from the stereotype we had of threesomes. It's a tender relationship."**

Some threesome arrangements come together around an existing couple, and that's one way of doing things. There is, of course, a second: The threesome could be made up of three people who have never had sex with each other but now wish to do so.

Beginning with a couple is riskier, because it has the potential to bring up feelings that may overwhelm the joy of the arrangement, such as jealousy or comparisons between oneself and another. The new member often takes the form of a gift. A man might allow another man into the bedroom because his companion wants to try a different kind of sex and he wants to help her realize this fantasy. But in doing so, he risks being forced into the background while she enjoys her present. Similarly, a woman may present her lover with a girl and may then become a bit of a third wheel as her man plays with his new toy.

How you put a threesome together is your business, but it is important to realize that the party could be wrecked if things unfold in this manner. Unless you enjoy being a monument to self-sacrifice, you may get hot under the collar rather than under the sheets as you watch your partner having fun with the new attraction rather than with you, especially if you had expected to be making love all together. Ideally, both of you will have sex with the new invitee. Making sure this happens will be a focus of future chapters.

Whatever your reasons for acting on your fantasies, if you're going to take the plunge, figure out how to do it right. If you're going ahead as a couple, you need to find a third. Josée Leboeuf, a clinical sexologist and psychotherapist from Quebec, provides some counsel:

> **"It's never easy to find someone [for a threesome], but there are a few methods. If you are thinking about someone, usually it's because he or she has shown signs of an open mind or because he or she has already had similar experiences. And if the person refuses, you must respect that choice without pressing for reasons. You also have to be clear on how far you are willing to go, and make [that] clear to your partner. Will you be able to look each other in the eye the next day? You have to talk over the acts that you don't want to perform, whether the three of you will spend the night together or not, etc. What will you do if you don't feel right? By planning ahead, you can make sure that you do feel right."**

To write this book I studied many situations involving multiple partners—my own experiences, stories in swingers magazines, and discussions on online sites—and I asked plenty of awkward questions. In the vast majority of cases, women seem to have ultimate authority over whether to share the sack with a third partner. This is true no matter whether the couple is inviting an extra man or woman: It is the woman who agrees to have another man in bed for her pleasure, or another woman for her lover's pleasure. She is the one who gives the green light for the couple to join an orgy.

In a way, this is a fine example of equality of the sexes in erotic matters. I suspect it also demonstrates a certain Machiavellian tendency in some men. They let their women bear sole responsibility for these decisions, even though they almost certainly steer their partners' choices, at least unconsciously. After all, bedding multiple partners is predominantly a male fantasy, as the polls discussed earlier suggest. So what can we conclude? Men almost always want sexual pleasures outside the norm, but are they weak-willed babies who have to ask their lovers/mothers for permission? Of course not. But allowing the woman to make the decision also has a certain amount of logic because women have more to lose should the adventure fail. They take psychological, social, and (if there's violence) even physical risks when participating in a threesome. So having both partners—but especially the woman—think things through before acting makes good sense.

How do you pick up a third partner? I don't need to spend much time answering this. It involves many of the same tactics as finding a first partner—mutual friends, flirting in a night club, the Internet. Below are a few thoughts from young women I know who have gotten into the act. "Why only women?" you might ask. Because, I believe, most guys don't talk about sex.

> **"One night after coming back from a club...we had a friend [stay] over—a guy who wanted to sleep off his drink for a couple of hours before driving home. Another friend—a girl—convinced us that it would be more fun if we all slept in the living room. The next morning there was underwear strewn all over the furniture."**

"It was a well thought-out decision, to have more and better sex, that led us to find a third partner who neither of us knew and who was easy to forget."

"[We were] with friends in a country house. I was having sex with my boyfriend in a tiny bedroom. He was lying on top of me when I saw one of our housemates checking us out at the door, laughing. I only needed to move a little to touch his leg, which I did. I put my naked foot on his fly. He happily took the bait, and a few minutes later his erect penis was between my breasts. My boyfriend had never been so surprised in his life."

"[This is the] true story of a three-way love affair, coupled with a large helping of homosexuality that was finally satisfied. I wanted to be with this girl, but I didn't want to leave my boyfriend. He was happy to adapt himself to the situation."

"Swingers clubs and X-rated films! The sight of group sex is almost banal, but I wanted to try it, and I had a chance, unexpectedly, with two guy friends who were always together. They had some homosexual tendencies, and my body was the only thing that could keep them apart—though not by much, since I'm so thin."

The Perfect Party For most guys and girls, making love with three, four, or more partners means that a long-held fantasy is going to come true. So it is important to remember that this might be your only shot. Here are a few simple ground rules to ensure success.

NO BRUSH-OFFS Once you've decided to plunge into lust and fornication together, everyone should have fun. Don't push anyone aside or make someone feel like a third wheel. It is especially critical not to brush off your regular partner. He or she will take that very badly. So when exploring nonmonogamous liaisons, you need to be able to manage and limit negative emotions. The two of you can do this together by:

- vowing a primary loyalty to your relationship
- limiting the intensity level when it comes to the other participant(s)
- promising there will be no emotional connection to other lovers
- practicing honesty at all times regarding your feelings

Honest, open communication beforehand also really helps, so seek to discuss topics like the following:

- Do you want a situation where one person watches the other two or will everyone be pleasured at the same time?
- Is pairing okay?
- What are your plans regarding safer sex?

NO BULLYING In some of the situations I will describe, one woman will be having sex with two or three men. This numerical advantage for the men should never lead to a situation suggesting rape, even if that plays a role in the fantasies of the woman offering herself to this group of horny men. Respect for her and sensitivity to her pleasure should be a constant.

Similarly, if one of the men has trouble with his erection—an understandable experience in such a new situation—the guys around him should not make a big deal out of it. The man who is briefly "out of order" still has a role to play: He can use his mouth, tongue, and fingers to pleasure the girl. Keeping the atmosphere relaxed will help him return to working order more quickly.

GIVE YOURSELVES SOME SPACE Having sex with two or three other people requires space. Some of the positions I will discuss—those that have the advantage of giving you something to boast about after—can only be performed on a bed that is three or four yards wide, like the ones they have in swingers clubs. So you'll have to prepare your place in advance or, if this is all happening on the spur of the moment, you'll have to be quick and resourceful. You can, for example, put a few mattresses down on the living room floor. For the party to take off, prepare your place according to the guidelines that libertines have been using for centuries.

- Dim the lights, but not too much. This kind of sex is meant to be seen.
- Set out something to drink for breaks. Champagne won't be wasted, but it can cause bad breath later on.
- Arrange some mirrors around the bed so that you can better see the actors.
- Put together a comfortable little corner in case someone needs a break and wants to continue watching the goings-on.

REMEMBER: SAFER SEX Finally, the most important rule of all: Everyone should stay safe by protecting their sexual health. The more partners involved and the more positions they try, the greater the risk for transmitting a variety of sexually transmitted infections (STIs). Throughout these pages, I will often pass on advice from the French organization called Couples

Contre le Sida (Couples Against AIDS). The basic rule is to use a new condom for each penetration of an orifice (vagina, anus, or mouth). A man who has unprotected vaginal or anal sex with two women one after the other, or who doesn't change condoms, runs the risk of transmitting infection. Of course, as in two-person sex, fiddling with condoms can cool the temperature, so you may want to turn the putting on of the condom into a game. And a couple who has been together for some time and has stopped using condoms will have to unwrap them again. This, too, can become part of the fun.

ADVICE FROM COUPLES AGAINST AIDS

Q: *What precautions should a partner take when performing oral sex on more than one person at a time?*

A: One should use a new latex (or polyurethane if you're allergic to latex) condom for each male and a new dental dam (or sheet of nonmicrowavable Saran Wrap) for every female. This diminishes the risks of infection, both for the person giving and for those receiving. Secretions infected with the HIV virus and other STIs can pass from the genitals of one person to another.

Q: *What precautions should a partner take when fingering multiple vaginas and anuses?*

A: Here again, it is best to avoid transmitting bodily fluids and germs from one entryway to another. One phrase you might remember is "one vagina: one finger," or "one anus: one finger." That is to say, use a different finger or fingers for each penetration. But since you only have ten fingers, you may need to use condoms, finger cots, or latex gloves (you still need to use different fingers for each penetration). If the gloves seem obtrusive you can trim them at the base of each finger, in effect making mini-condoms. Don't forget to trim your fingernails so that they don't rip the barrier method you are using.

Q: *What about for penetrating different partners?*

A: When penetrating several partners in succession, you should change condoms after each one so that vaginal or anal secretions don't get mixed together and HIV or other infections are not transmitted. The person doing the penetration can infect his multiple partners without their knowing it, even though, in using protection, he himself is not high risk for acquiring HIV. Men are often asymptomatic, but women who participate in sex with multiple partners regularly complain of contracting STIs. If a relation is just between two people but vaginal penetration follows anal penetration, changing condoms is still crucial because vaginal infection can result from the transmission of bacteria from the anus to the vagina.

AND FINALLY, KEEP A CODE OF SILENCE! Even as you are having fun, think about the next day. You've had an extravagant experience, but it would not be a good idea to tell everyone and his mother about it. No one will come away unharmed if your little secret is divulged. That's why, when choosing a lover for multiple partner sex, it is important to find someone who is not only attractive but also discreet.

Those are the rules, folks. You see—it is not that complicated.

ch 2. One Guy, Two Girls

Triophilia: The desire to form a sexual triangle with three partners, usually two females and one male, and aiming to fulfill the bisexual desires of all members.

— *Nouveau dictionnaire de sexologie*
(The New Dictionary of Sexology)

One guy and two girls—a man's favorite fantasy finally comes true.

There are plenty of ways you can get there. A lady friend jumps in bed with the couple, a friendly evening takes a surprising turn, you meet on the Internet or at a nightclub exit. This book starts with what happens once the threesome gets home. We accompany them on their search for shared pleasure, which is hopefully divided equally among the three participants.

Let's begin by exploring the case of a little adventure in which everyone is strictly heterosexual. A later chapter, "The Perfect Triangle," may make them regret that they've limited their pleasure to the opposite sex.

The Bustling Threesome The 1967 dictionary quoted in the epigraph asserts that a sexual embrace between three people can only occur when one is bisexual. Maybe. But I'm going to focus on the guy who is completely heterosexual—and a lucky devil.

IT IS NOT THAT SIMPLE A naked guy between two women who are making love to him. This is the fantasy of the harem, very popular among men. But when it is about to happen, guys sometimes panic. This is understandable because it feels dangerous. Every man worries about his reputation—how he'll do—when trying to satisfy two women simultaneously. From his point of view he simply must perform. His masculinity is on the line.

"How should a man act when he's with two women?" That's what the French magazine *Max* addresses in its article, "Have Sex with Two Women":

> "First off, it's best not to be too boastful. The women outnumber you in this situation, and they can easily make fun of you if you play at being macho. When it comes to love and sex, women often call the shots—don't forget that! If you're the shy type, you're probably well off in this situation. The two girls can excite you with hot looks; they can arouse you to the core by making love right in front of you. The idea is that they pet each other, rub against you, embrace you one after the other and then at the same time. As for you, you should divide your attention and kisses equally. If it works, you've hit the jackpot. After all, threesomes exponentially increase the potential for pleasure."

TO BEGIN, A BATH Ideally, the bathtub is the place to start the night, as long as it is big enough. A shower stall can also work well, but you have to make the narrowness work to your advantage. Having sex with a new partner always requires learning about his or her body, and when there are two new partners, you have twice the work. Some saunas catering to swingers have figured out how well the shower does this—they organize their stalls so that everyone can see everyone else. Being naked together facilitates everything that follows. You can relax and get comfortable with one anothers' bodies and with the situation.

The shower also gives you an innocent excuse to start stroking each other because you can soap one anothers' bodies. First, the girls wash the guy's intimate parts, so they can be sure they will be tasting a clean penis. They can take advantage of the situation by feeling him up. The man, for his part, can slide a washcloth into the clefts of the ladies' behinds and finish cleaning them by hand.

The most difficult thing is resisting the urge to begin having sex right there, in the water. The little shower stall has everything you need for lovemaking. Bodies covered in soap slip-slide easily against each other, wet kisses can go back and forth, and hands that linger on breasts can give all the pleasure one needs.

Plus, showering together has another big advantage: You can be sure everyone will be clean. The person who invites the other two into his or her bed can even choose soaps with scents that are a turn-on (ginger soap, in particular, has a reputation as an aphrodisiac). After all this initial attention, you'll have more confidence in your body and in your friends' bodies, too. And it is more than a question of hygiene. Sucking on the genitals or anus of a man or woman with whom you have just showered—and whose body you have just caressingly washed—is a lot easier than getting into bed with a stranger.

A SAFER SEX SOLUTION—THE FEMALE CONDOM

A regular condom isn't the best option when you're with more than one woman. So whenever girls outnumber guys—two girls, one guy, for example—using female condoms is a must. The female condom, sometimes also called a "femidom" or "femidon," is a marvelous invention with many advantages for your little threesome. The guy, going from one woman to the other—or, to be precise, from one vagina to the next—doesn't have to change condoms each time. This will keep the experience hotter for everyone. If only one woman wears a condom, the man should put one on when penetrating the other woman, unless she is his regular partner and they choose not to use this type of protection. (Note that a male condom should not be used with a female condom as this increases the risk of tearing.) If you don't have a female condom, the guy has to change condoms after every penetration. Remember that anal sex also demands a condom.

Another advantage of using a female condom: Putting it in place can be fun in its own right. First, make sure the lady's vagina is wet—a fingertip touch can check it out. Then, put in the condom using two fingers to slide it in. If you do your job well, you may very well elicit a little groan of pleasure.

THE ERECTION: A LITTLE PROBLEM Any guy can tell you this—there's a principle that arises at the intersection of math, psychology, and physiology: The more partners a guy entertains, the greater the risk that he will leave them unsatisfied, either because he can't get it up or because he comes too quickly. Yet the circumstances demand a virtuoso performance.

The French-Canadian website www.canoe.com, contains a section called "Art de vivre" (The Art of Living) that gives a good description of the dangers guys run up against.

> **"Guys also feel reticent, even if the majority of them would never dare admit it. [Although] in their waking fantasies they are inexhaustible stallions who can keep a harem moaning all night, in real life, many are worried about their actual capacity. It is not rare that Jules ducks out when Julie (surprise!) agrees to a threesome."**

By way of illustration, the website narrates the misadventure of Marc, a twenty-seven-year-old computer technician, who had another problem, just as bad:

> **"My fiancée at the time, her best friend, and I were lying on the bed, talking. Then I noticed they were stroking each other in a way that was more than friendly. I was aroused, but when I saw them kissing, I totally blew it. Like an ass, I ejaculated before the party could even get started."**

It might be useful to take some advice from the experts. Ejaculation can be controlled, and the longer a man can keep his erection, the better he can prolong the pleasure of his two partners. Chinese philosophers suggest taking a few minutes off when the ejaculation feels as if it is about to happen. Contemporary sexologists say that you should squeeze the penis around the glans (the tip) to prevent a soon-to-come ejaculation. That's also the technique porn stars use.

◎ **Who's Who?** Who comes over will play a major role in determining how your night turns out. The atmosphere will be different depending on whether you're all strangers—sexually speaking—or if two of you are everyday partners.

A COUPLE AND THEIR LADY FRIEND This is definitely the most common configuration, even if I don't have the statistics to prove it. A couple decides to spice up their sex life by adding the charms of another woman. The man in this adventure is lucky indeed! His lover has agreed to intimacies that morality generally condemns: She's about to let another woman slide into your bed, and supposedly without hoping for pleasure of her own, since she isn't attracted to her own sex.

Men, you must be up to the task. And, above all, you have to be sure that your girlfriend is as happy with the results as you are. What motivates a completely heterosexual woman to take this step might seem mysterious. She wants to give her boyfriend a gift—but that can't be all, unless it is because she doesn't feel she is good enough in bed. More likely, she wants to satisfy a fantasy of her own: She may want to play with another woman or even act the voyeur and watch you have sex with someone else. No matter what her motivation, the experience can certainly satisfy her curiosity and, hopefully, will excite her as well. Your job is simple: Make her come like never before. The night should be organized, even staged, so that her fantasy becomes a joyful reality.

THE THIRD: A PLAYTHING FOR THE COUPLE? Didier, a young man I met on the Internet, compares the role of the third partner with the position of a married man's mistress. Existing outside the bonds of matrimony, the mistress has the advantage of being free from sentimental attachment. "She comes over when she wants to and has sex when she wants to. She doesn't have to be there for the hard times or be involved in arguments because the couple treats her as a plaything. She's a special kind of friend; [one who] can inject herself into the couple and become almost family. But she can also leave when she likes." Didier adds, "The downsides to this situation? There are plenty. Everything you would imagine to be bad, is bad. But you have that in any living situation, so...." Didier's voice trails off.

(As my more clever readers may have already realized, the names of interviewees for this book have been changed so that they all begin with A, B, C, and D. Aside from protecting their reputations, this allows me to describe triangles and other complicated figures more easily.)

THE PERFECT EVENING

Ari and Béatrice have talked about it for weeks, maybe even months. Now, the day is here and they have managed to persuade Carla to join them. How did they do it? That's their business. Maybe Ari came on to her, or maybe it was Béatrice. Perhaps they met her in a nightclub or swingers club, or found her in the classifieds. How they did it is not the focus here.

Ari greets Carla at his and Béatrice's place. All three have a drink together, and, as they talk, Béatrice remains a bit distant—she's warm and cheerful, but she lets Ari and Carla develop a connection. As Ari begins to kiss Carla, Béatrice stays to the side, even though she watches every movement. Carla could be put off by Béatrice's attitude, but she quickly figures out what's going on. As if she's at the theater, Béatrice is settled comfortably in a chair or lying on the bed; she begins rubbing her breasts and sliding a hand into her wet panties. Before joining in, she wants to enjoy watching. Béatrice's fantasy may have a narcissistic component to it: Watching Ari have sex with another woman might allow her to imagine herself making love to him. That's one possibility, anyway.

What *is* certain is that, pretty soon, Béatrice can't hold out any longer. As soon as Carla is finished, Béatrice pulls Ari away and takes Carla's place. Now Ari has to "give 110 percent," as sports magazines put it. Sure, he ejaculated a few minutes ago in Carla's vagina, but now he has to get hard again and perform with more gusto than ever. Béatrice is expecting a moment hot with pleasure. Luckily for Ari, she's wet enough that it doesn't take her long to come, which allows him to save a little strength for what's coming next. This was just the appetizer. Now both girls are satisfied, and they are ready to go on to the main course—a real threesome. Ari, tired but exhilarated, will be the guest of honor.

That's how it is supposed to work. But many couples trying a threesome leave with less-than-pleasant memories. It doesn't take much for everything to fall apart—a whiff of jealousy, a pinch of frustration. If the female half of the couple gets less pleasure from the situation than she expected, the whole thing risks leaving a bitter taste in her mouth. And a bitter taste in her mouth is a bitter taste in his mouth.

A FIASCO

"I had been living with Annie for a few months, sleeping in her bed in an apartment she shared with Chantal. One night we came back from an odd job that the three of us did for the local bus company, and Annie began to flirt with Chantal quite openly. She suggested that I take them both to bed. This was during the hippie era, when things like that seemed perfectly natural. We settled into a bed in an alcove off the main hallway. The beginning of the night was wonderful for me. I'd fantasized about seeing Chantal naked, and I was not disappointed. She was thin, delicate, and her little, white breasts—almost adolescent—enthralled me. I immediately began to touch them, to bite them, while Annie lay down and let her ample chest press against Chantal's back. She began rubbing against Chantal's body and begging Chantal to stroke her. But I was only interested in Chantal, and I started to bang her without a single gesture, a single acknowledgment that Annie was there—and she became a spectator to a catastrophe that she herself had

engineered.... Chantal probably thought I was a brute as I slid in and out of her tight vagina without much care.... But we managed to come together, or at least she let me think we did. And when we returned to reality, we were alone in bed. Annie was pretending to sleep, and the night no longer had any erotic ecstasy at all." – David

THREE LOVERS, TOGETHER FOR THE VERY FIRST TIME

In this situation, no one needs to worry about the ongoing relationship of the couple. The three lovers are on an equal footing, no one has an axe to grind, and no one will have to say afterward, "Of course I still love you, I love only you." The guy, still alone with two girls, at least has one less thing to worry about, which should help him relax a bit.

So on an emotional level, this situation is a lot easier to manage than one built around a couple. The trio is interested in exploring sex together and for pleasure—and have no ulterior motives that might derail the evening. There are no couples, no jealousy, no suspicions to keep at bay. All anyone wants is to try out the moves, positions, words, and situations that drive pleasure together. I'll explore these in a moment.

If the threesome turns into an out-of-bed affair, things might become complicated. But that's for another book—and it is the subject of most of the films I recommend at the end of this book.

◎ **The Kama Su'Trois** When three lovers have sex all together—as opposed to pairs just taking turns—they have a large number of positions to choose from. Many are acrobatic; all are wonderful to see and do. It is hard for even a guidebook like this to give readers a sense of how much fun group experiences can be, but you will feel the pleasures firsthand as you go along.

The sex scene illustrated in Figure 2.1, which is by French illustrator Martin Van Maële, frankly demonstrates one of the ways you can begin your evening. A young man sits between two girls. Both girls have their legs spread, and each has hooked one of her thighs over one of his legs, allowing him access to their private areas. He has his hands full. He strokes both of them, feeling his way through their lace petticoats. One of the girls, meanwhile, has taken his erect penis in her hand and is vigorously playing with it. From the look of the image, all of this is just the beginning for this threesome.

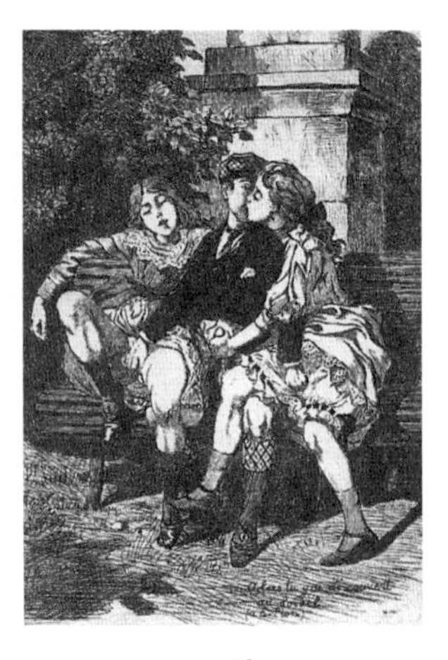

FIGURE 2.1. ***Alors tu y as été souvent au bordel?* (So, you've been often to the brothel?) from *La Grande danse macabre des vifs* (The Grand Macabre Dance of the Dead) (from Wikimedia Commons, the free media repository)**

THE LITTLE KING HAS FUN

In a threesome, a man can enjoy one of those moments that he might recall forever as one of his best erotic experiences. He can watch the two women taking turns kissing his penis as he stands or kneels (see Figure 2.2). As one girl kisses him, the other slides her tongue down to his testicles and starts to lick them, kiss them, and take them in her mouth. Guys, are you getting excited? If you are, remember this caveat: This delightful maneuver is so titillating that it should be reserved for moments when even the most virile man is exhausted and needs something to get him back up. Use it at any other time, and Ari might come in someone's mouth before the fun even gets started.

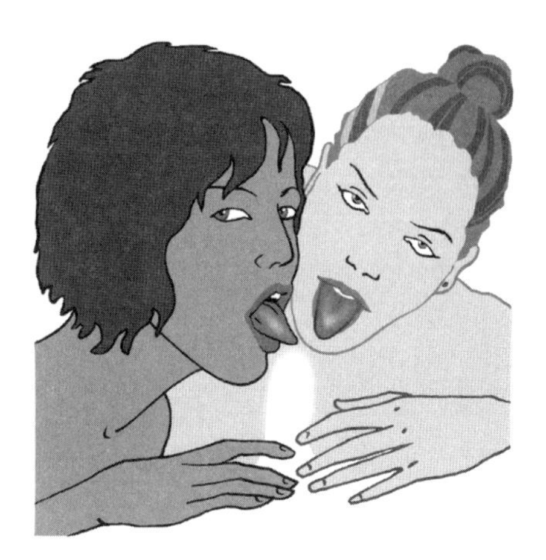

FIGURE 2.2. **Daring to explore your sexuality with multiple partners can take you to new levels of pleasure—while simultaneously allowing you to play out long-held fantasies.**

Everyone should take advantage of what a threesome offers beyond what's possible with two people in a bed. Let's take a second to dwell on a threesome scene that you've probably seen many times in X-rated movies. For both women, fellatio practiced together should be first of all a cooperative effort, not a competition. Carla and Béatrice can go back and forth between two different positions. Sometimes one of them will work alone, and sometimes the two will work together.

Carla carefully watches Béatrice sucking off Ari, watching from different angles. One moment, she moves in closer, the next, she has settled farther away. She doesn't want to miss anything. Usually a woman doesn't see much when sucking off a guy—maybe some hair that's going into her nose, or a close-up of the guy's lower abs. And mirrors are no help unless she wants a stiff neck. So this threesome gives Carla a chance to see a man's penis up close, to observe how it quivers with pleasure when a woman's mouth takes hold of its tip, to watch how it trembles as excitement mounts, and also to see what a girl looks like while she performs fellatio. "Are you kidding? My mouth is open that wide? My lips stretch that much? No wonder I get cramps."

Of course, the woman watching need not feel left out. She can find ways to pleasure other parts of the man's body. For example, she can stroke his thighs or play with his testicles. For this scene to be a dream come true, both girls have to keep touching Ari throughout.

Sometimes, Béatrice and Carla combine their efforts. The most difficult part of playing together is to avoid bumping heads as the two explore their little king's penis. They can try dividing it up—having two mouths on one penis allows the ladies to suck or kiss two different sections of one of the most sensitive parts of the man's body. The penis is actually one immense pleasure organ, from the testicles to the glans (the tip).

The duet can take several forms. Béatrice can suck Ari's glans while Carla rolls his testicles around in her mouth. The two of them can both kiss the stem of his penis, or one can lick his anus—rimming the lucky guy—while the other keeps working on his member. And why only play with the lower half? While one woman continues on that erect organ, the other can kiss him on the mouth or nibble at his erect nipples.

LYING DOWN: 69 PLUS Double fellatio can also work when the man is too tired to sit or stand. While he lies on his back, one of the girls takes advantage to get a little treat for herself. She sits on top of his mouth, putting herself in a 69 position, while the other lady kneels down between his legs. Everybody gives each other oral pleasure. The girls can trade places so they both get a chance to enjoy his oral services. A little later, one of them skewers herself with his penis, which is nice and hard after all of the attention. And this brings us to another position: the two horsewomen.

THE TWO HORSEWOMEN This is one of those extravagant configurations you can only try with three playful lovers. The guy lies on his back and one of the girls sits on his face, allowing him to lick and kiss her vagina. The second girl straddles the guy's hips and begins having sex with him. But be careful. You don't want him asphyxiated and crushed—that would ruin the fun. The two gals have to be gentle, and they must be light.

Will this satisfy everyone? Not necessarily. The woman riding the guy's face is most likely to come, while the man, crushed under everyone's weight, will have a hard time focusing on pleasuring himself with that butt and wet vagina masking his face. Unless...well, unless he can make himself feel that his tongue and erect penis are part of the same organ. Once he can convince himself of that—that he has two penises with which to satisfy two ladies—he'll be on the way to making an incredible fantasy come true. Now that's an art. To really bring the fantasy to life, he'll have to be an active participant, taking hold of the butt resting on his face and helping it move. He'll have to take charge of the situation, at least to some degree, and do more than simply submit to being a bench.

THE CANDLESTICK How else can a man use his tongue and penis at the same time? A user of the site www.aufeminin.com offers an idea: "The boy sits, legs wide for better balance.

The smaller girl penetrates herself with his penis, and the two of them embrace as she crouches on him. They form a candlestick—only the candle is missing." The larger woman, standing, straddles her two lovers and puts her stomach and vagina up against the face of the young man, awaiting his tongue, while the other girl feels up her butt, perhaps even licking her behind. Of course, depending on her tastes, the girl who's standing also can offer her vagina to her female partner (see Figure 2.3).

In this position and others, the woman not at the center of the action must take care not to turn into a piece of furniture. She can't do much as the second girl sits on her and enjoys the guy's kisses, penetrations, and whatever other desires possess him. By leaning back on the headboard and serving as a pillow, the girl who has become a spectator can give her female counterpart a place to stay as the guy does his work. She gives her friend the wonderful feeling of being curled up in a big cushion of soft, heaving flesh.

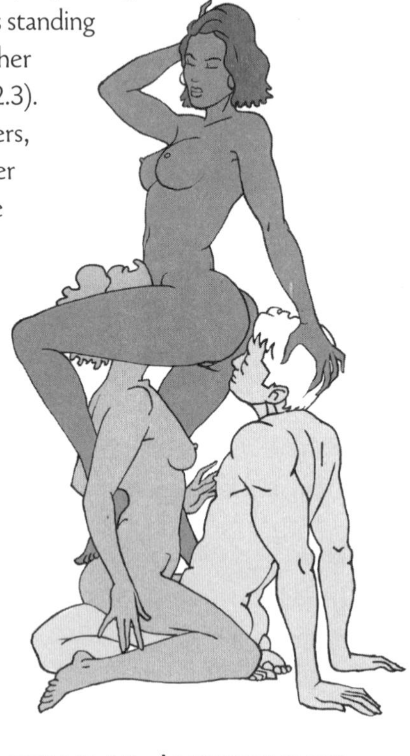

FIGURE 2.3. **An openness to new positions and techniques—such as the Candlestick position illustrated here—are key to exploring multiple-partner experiences.**

The girl who is out of the action gets compensated, though. She can watch the performance and get pleasure of a different kind: vicarious.

TO EACH HER DUE The two women both slide female condoms into their wet vaginas. The guy is going to penetrate them one after the other, and he'll try to satisfy them both. How vigorously he moves will play a large part in getting the girls excited. But even more important will be how they manage the frustration that can accompany seeing a lover leave for another woman and then return. As many couples have discovered, anticipation can be one of the best parts of sex. To get the most out of the man's back-and-forth, wait until the foreplay has raised the women's arousal to fever pitch. This way, as the male lover enjoys the other girl, the spectator will have plenty of incentive to stroke herself and wait expectantly.

The two girls can be on their hands and knees, their bodies parallel. Or they can lie on their backs, so that the guy can see their beautiful faces and bodies. What's most important is that the guy can go back and forth quickly—and that his moves excite his lovers. Who will come first? Will they come together, or will he come with only one of them? Whatever the conclusion, it is important to take it all in stride. While it may not end with all three coming together, there can still be a very happy ending.

Other positions for this configuration require a bit more bisexuality on the part of the ladies—I'll get into those later in a chapter called "The Perfect Triangle."

HOW WAS IT? Alan, a twenty-seven-year-old bartender from Montreal, is an aficionado of threesomes. He's happy to answer that much-asked question: How was it?

"It's so great to be kissed by one woman while another one is giving you fellatio. And to watch two beauties stroke each other and get pleasure from each other is also fabulous. But I especially love the buzz that you get when you make two girls come at the same time, or when you and a guy friend make a girl come like she never has before."

Someone had to say it.

ch 3. One Girl, Two Guys

Trioïsm: Coitus between two people, men or women, watched by a third, who sometimes takes part in the coitus. This sexual practice tends to satisfy voyeurs, homosexuals, and exhibitionists. When there are more than three people, the proper terminology is *group sexuality*.

—*Dictionnaire de l'amour, de l'érotisme, et de la sexualité*
(Dictionary of Love, Erotica, and Sexuality)

In this chapter, as in the last, we will explore situations involving three hetero partners. In "The Perfect Triangle," the next chapter, we focus on threesomes involving bisexual partners—which are a lot more fun, I think.

Double the Pleasure Didier, the guy we met on the Internet, explains:

"A trio involves a couple, whether married or not, and a third partner. It's not an orgy, because there are rules you have to follow. In general, the husband or boyfriend wants to create a trio with two men and one woman. He uses his wife to fulfill

a latent homosexual desire that he won't even admit to himself."

In this little description we see a common prejudice regarding the MMF threesome—that the man "uses his wife" to satisfy his own homosexual inclinations.

But of course that isn't the whole story. Is it so difficult to imagine that a woman might want to be touched, held, kissed, and made love to by two men? That she might want to find out for herself what this feels like?

For an adventurous and voluptuous young woman, this can be a very thrilling experience. A woman daring enough to try this will discover a treasure trove of joy—as long as her lovers aren't self-absorbed morons. That's the most important thing to avoid. The guys she chooses should be focused on more than their own gratification; they need to be as interested—more interested, really—in giving her a good time. And they must understand that they are getting into a situation that requires tact and charm.

A FANTASY? Many women's magazines treat having sex with two guys as a fantasy to be analyzed, instead of a desire to be acted upon. Take a look at this article by Julia Rambal, "*Ce que révèlent nos fantasmes*" (What Our Fantasies Tell Us):

"The fantasy of having multiple partners satisfies our desire to lose ourselves. We are no longer in an intimate situation, and we can express ourselves freely. The fantasy reveals a desire for fierce sex that takes us far beyond convention. We become the object of pleasure, enjoyed by the hands, tongues, and genitals of men. We feel that our bodies are completely full. This fantasy also

reveals a secret desire to be so sexy that no one can resist our charms.

"There is a variant: fantasizing about sleeping with the best friend of your boyfriend. This doesn't mean that you want to cheat on your lover. Rather, it suggests that you want more control over his life, because you're worried that he's going to run away from you. In this case, the fantasy suggests a lack of confidence in yourself."

The article then goes on to ask:

"[S]hould you take the plunge? A fantasy has one advantage: You can decide on the screenplay. In reality, your partner may not react as expected. Your bodies won't move as you'd imagined. It's up to you. But it's best not to suggest this to your regular lover: He may not like the idea of sharing you at all."

Unfortunately, this way of thinking about women's fantasies of threesomes represents the status quo. People—women included—dismiss their fantasies by labeling them as subconscious desires for loss of control, fierce sex, control over sexuality, and the wish to be the center of attention. And they don't act on them.

WHO ARE THEY? Anna Rozen, in her book of short stories, *Plaisir d'offrir, joie de reçevoir* (The Pleasure of Giving, the Joy of Receiving), notes:

"There's just one difficulty in creating the ideal threesome, the ideal trio to preside over: I have to have the right partners. It's impossible to do

this right just any day, with a boyfriend and his best friend, or, for that matter, with your best friend. The two of them have probably never seen each other under the right circumstances. I've never known my partners in threesomes very well. Doing this with friends is not really possible. Threesomes require some mystery, something unknown; no experience, no memory or fear should trouble the simple combination of flesh and desire. I've never been able to figure out how the guys in a threesome relate to each other. Are they like friends who get together once a week to play tennis?"

SETTING UP THE DREAM Foreplay between two lovers can be wild, but when there are three, it becomes downright wicked. The two guys should forget about their own pleasure and focus on giving the girl what she wants—all of the touches and sensations that she fantasized about while singing her Siren's song and roping her suitors into bed. Working together, the guys should caress and stimulate her until the poor thing is about to faint. Or they can take on opposite roles: One plays at being rough, biting and spanking her, while the other is tender, petting and kissing her.

Here is one position that will do everything she dreams of: One guy takes care of her below, giving her a good, long cunnilingus; meanwhile, the second guy plays with her upper body, kissing her on the mouth and playing with her breasts. Here's another position the girl can take advantage of: She can enjoy both cunnilingus and rimming at the same time—the clit and the anus can both be in on the fun. Of course, the guys might want to use their fingers, too—and this can lead to a whole different sort of double penetration.

There are gentler strokes, too—massages and soft touches. But unless you want the afternoon to be more like a spa session than a sex session, these will have to give way to more sexual strokes, themselves the signals of even better things to come. Why not prepare ahead of time by putting out a little bottle of massage oil?

SAFER SEX: CONDOMS A-GO-GO Don't start an adventure such as this one without a big box of condoms—a dozen is probably the bare minimum. By the end, the floor could be covered in crumpled latex.

Choreographing the Action There are two ways a male-male-female (MMF) threesome can play out: The guys can go one after the other, or they can work together. Either way, the threesome will be a rare experience, and you should take advantage of every minute. The tone of what follows sounds a bit like a workout video. I apologize for that. Just remember: This is about having fun!

ONE AFTER THE OTHER Having the guys go one after the other is the simpler way to run this threesome. A girl has sex with one guy while the other looks on, then it is the second guy's turn, and then she is back to the first guy. Put like that, it doesn't sound all that exciting, but in practice it can be, as Anita will tell you. She's been in a regular threesome for a few months. "My favorite positions aren't the ones where all three of us are tossing around together," Anita explains. "Sure, sometimes we melt into a big heap of thighs and chests. But then there are moments where I feel like the pleasure will never end—those are my favorite. My two friends are big voyeurs. That's good, because they spend a lot of their time looking and waiting while I have sex with the other. I know it's terrible of me to say it, but I like making them wait. All the positions help vary the kind of pleasure I get, and they keep the guy who is watching excited. While having sex, I also keep in mind my voyeur's pleasure. The performance I give has to be my best, it has to be beautiful and tight, so that he'll want to come over and have sex with me next. Because when I'm in these situations, I really want to be taken without pause."

Do all guys like this? Probably not. On the same website where I met Anita, a guy said he was skeptical that a heterosexual guy could enjoy this. "I've tried threesomes with two guys and one girl twice. ... I'm not homosexual enough—I'm not homosexual at all, actually—and so I don't find this any more fun than a night with my girlfriend and an X-rated film. I don't get much out of it. But she does, obviously!"

I should add one important note here: Sex with two guys can make the men competitive: Who will make her come harder and longer? Which one will have sex with her more often? However much they may boast of their sexual prowess, the guys now have to put up or shut up. The three partners, whether they gather together on the spur of the moment or plan this adventure in advance, have to have a sense of humor about this natural competitiveness or it'll spoil the fun.

IN IT TOGETHER Nature, in her great wisdom, endowed woman with three beautiful orifices, all of them beguiling to look at and fun to explore—and guys can explore each of these with their penises. These orifices are, of course, the vagina, the mouth, and the anus. A woman also has two hands, and even two breasts—all of which she can use to stroke the men's erections.

A threesome allows the girl to offer these charms to her men. One guy can take hold of the girl while the other strokes her, kisses her, or does whatever else he likes—perhaps he tickles and pinches her.

IS SHE A FINGER TRAP?

Guys, watch out! A threesome may be a bit trickier than you think—at least if you believe in the power of humorous slang to hide a deep truth. A Chinese finger trap is a small woven-straw cylinder sold at fairs and novelty shops that traps you if you insert a finger in each end. The harder you struggle, the tighter the trap holds. Supposedly, Asian police used these to restrain prisoners. But the phrase Chinese finger trap can also refer to a woman who has sex with two men at the same time. Does this mean that she could trap two guys together forever? It is worth thinking about.

LIGHTING TWO CANDLES AT ONCE Fellating two guys at once is no easy task. Oddly, doing it right is all in the gaze and the hand. As the girl sucks off one guy, she has to put on a good show for the guy she's momentarily abandoning. She should keep his penis in her hand and shoot him looks that keep him involved and show that she still cares.

Another thing: Don't play out this adventure like they do in those grotesque and often humiliating X-rated movie scenes: The men stand awkwardly with their hands dangling; the girl is on her knees at their feet. Instead, find positions that keep all three of you comfortable. The two guys can lie side-by-side; if the girl is on her knees between them she can easily reach and give pleasure to both. She may also try this facing away from the men, showing off her heavenly bottom as she first kisses one guy's sex and then the other's. This position may make the eye-games more difficult, but it has its own advantages. This way, the guys will be able to play with her ass and everything else they can find.

And there's still another way. The girl can take both penises in her mouth at the same time—or at least try to. Unfortunately, this is possible only if the penises are small. From the guy's perspective, it might be better if this doesn't work.

FRONT AND BACK Anita is on her knees, sucking off Brian, while Charles takes her doggy style (see Figure 3.1). This is a

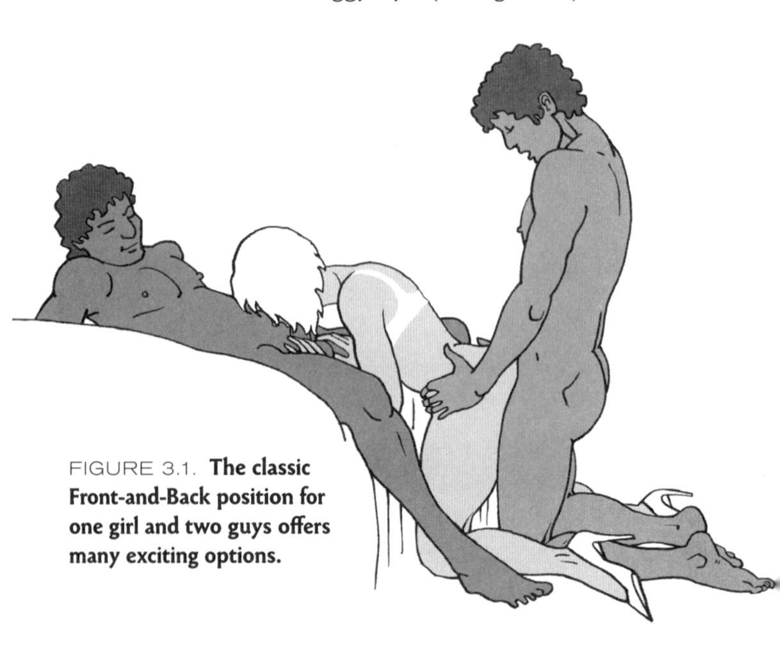

FIGURE 3.1. **The classic Front-and-Back position for one girl and two guys offers many exciting options.**

classic position, so what can I add? Well, there are the variations. Brian can get on his knees facing Anita and stroke her breasts, or he can lie down beneath her on his back, which allows Anita to lie down when she gets tired. He can lie with his head near her vagina, in a 69 position, giving him a courtside view of Charles penetrating Anita, or he can sit on a bed or a chair while Anita is on all fours on the floor. Finally, he can stand up facing her, which forces Anita to lift her torso and arch her ass—something Charles will surely like. Obviously, he can try anal penetration, too.

Another variation: Anita lies on a table, flat on her stomach, which puts her vagina and mouth at the proper height for this game. This position often receives crude attention from porn directors and, as a result, it has lost some of its eroticism and all of its romance. But for women who are willing to try it, I promise some unforgettable moments.

Anita will find it difficult to concentrate simultaneously on the pleasure she's getting and the pleasure she's giving. She also has to think about keeping her balance. If she doesn't, and Charles thrusts too hard, she might dive forward onto Brian's penis.

INDIAN SWING Yves Ferroul, a sexologist, described this position, which you can see on bas-relief sculptures from India, in her book *La sexualité féminine* (Female Sexuality):

> **"Two men stand face to face, holding up a woman between them. Her back is pointing to the floor and her stomach to the ceiling, her legs are around one man's shoulders, while he holds her by her ass so that her vulva touches his penis; she lets her shoulders push against the other**

man's chest as he holds her by the small of the back and plays with her stomach and breasts. Meanwhile, she strokes his penis."

Athletic types will especially appreciate positions like this one, which allow one man to carry the girl while the other penetrates her. They can finally use all those muscles they're so proud of.

GREEK SEX Actresses in X-rated films call this double vaginal penetration—two penises penetrate the vagina at the same time. Obviously, this requires a vagina that's big, well lubricated, and—most important—wants it. According to the *Encyclopedia of Unusual Sex Practices* by Brenda Love, this is a "Greek" practice.

THE SANDWICH, OR DOUBLE PENETRATION This ritual, known as the sandwich, is almost required in porn films. A woman is taken in both the vagina and the anus at once—she is the filling of the sandwich. The bread? The two men, of course. This position got its name soon after the sandwich (the food item, that is) was invented in the mid-eighteenth century.

Note that penetrating the vagina and the anus at the same time is not easy. As Didier, our friend from the Internet forum for threesomes fans, says: "As to double penetration, which women in threesomes are sometimes willing to try, making it work is not always easy. The two men only have a few ways of going about it. The positions aren't comfortable, and the men might get cramps. Moreover, for both men to come at the same time the girl does, you have to synchronize two ejaculations—that's hard. The three partners have to be very much in sync, which means they have to already have experience together." Do you really have to ejaculate together? Can't one guy come after the other? Maybe that's all right, as long as the first man to finish stays in her until she comes. You don't want to deprive the girl of the incredible sensation just as she's coming to her peak.

The hardest part of this position, however, is not the coming together; it is the preparing. The woman's vaginal membranes are fragile, and two penises together could potentially hurt them. Anal sex alone needs a lot of preparation—first a lubricant and then long stretching and relaxing. In the heat of the moment, two guys might miss even the most elementary caresses, especially since a large member in the vagina makes anal penetration even more difficult. You really need to prep the anus for these penetrations. A nice water-based lubricant combined with a tender finger or two to relax the anal sphincter should do it. And, as you know, taking care of oneself and one's partner is an important part of double penetration: The men must don those nice, little condoms.

There aren't a lot of great positions for this meaty sandwich, and it is even harder to find one that all three partners will enjoy. I recommend a few possibilities below.

STANDING UP Standing up is probably the easiest position, although all partners have to be about the same height. The gal stands between the two guys. The man in front holds one of her legs up to make penetrating her vagina easier. She holds onto this guy's torso, while the one who is about to have anal sex with her grabs her hips. Everyone can move back and forth. The two men can thrust together or in counterpoint, in any rhythm they like. Either way, she will have the lovely sensation of being completely full. When her knees buckle and she slides to the floor, drunk on joy or fatigue, her beaus must catch her.

LYING DOWN The three partners lie on the side of the bed, letting their legs wind together, as in Figure 3.2 below. The lady, who seems so comfortable here, opens her legs wide and points them up to the ceiling. The two guys, equally at ease, can play with the girl's ass, breasts, thighs, and hips—all the while going as deep into her as they want.

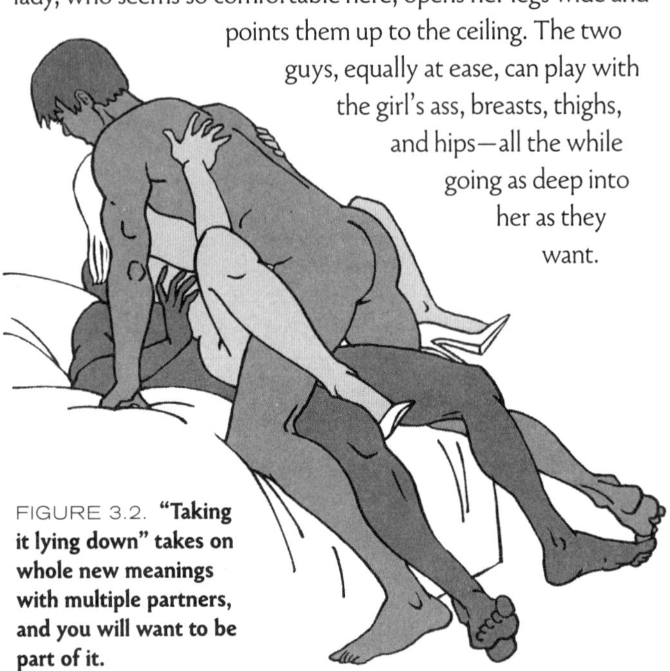

FIGURE 3.2. **"Taking it lying down" takes on whole new meanings with multiple partners, and you will want to be part of it.**

THE AMAZONIAN One guy lies on his back and the lady straddles him. He slips his penis in and begins to explore her vagina. Then comes the second guy, sliding behind and taking advantage of her butt. In porn films, this is the position most commonly used for the sandwich.

LITERATURE INSPIRED BY DOUBLE PENETRATION Here are just a few snippets of literature inspired by double penetration:

"When I was eighteen, maybe nineteen, I was in two or three sandwiches.... My boyfriend, a fan of [the soccer team] Paris Saint-Germain, had friends who were kind of cute. There was only one problem: They always wanted to keep their sweaty jerseys on, even in bed.... Also, they only seemed to know twenty-four words. Since they knew how to say *asshole* in four different languages, that left them twenty words with which they could ask me what I wanted in bed."
—Linux, Elsa, *Le Journal d'Elsa Linux* (Elsa Linux's Diary)

"Our penises were no longer very hard, but we took her in a sandwich anyway, in order to have regular sex and anal sex with her at the same time. We hadn't done this yet and wanted to be able to say we had. I was in her cunt, and André was behind. He came very quickly, with a little feminine moan—the result, undoubtedly, of being tired. He'd screwed her three times. I stopped screwing her a little later, since I'd already come twice and at my age, you shouldn't ask too much of Mr. Johnson. Zaza didn't come either, but even as she finished, exhausted, her desire sated, I could tell that she had liked it and that she would remember this experience during later encounters." —Esparbec, *Les Main baladeuses* (Wandering Hands)

"The abbess who was found in the company of two monks received the attentions of a sergeant and a corporal. Naturally, the sergeant, being the superior officer, went first. He threw himself on the bed and tried to pull the abbess toward him. At first she resisted, but the corporal, who had his own plan, gave her a push in the sergeant's direction. The superior officer seized her immediately and pushed his member in so hard that she couldn't withhold a deep sigh. When the corporal—following his plan—saw that the sergeant was giving her a good screw, he took his cock in his hand and pushed it in behind. The poor abbess, she wasn't expecting that treachery. She tried to flee from his unexpected attack, but she managed only to run herself through on the sergeant's penis. He responded with a thrust so hard that the corporal felt it. Back and forth the abbess went, and she wound up feeling the sting of pleasure."

— Anonymous, *Les Pucelages conquis* (Conquered Virginity)

"D.P., for deep penetration, is the name we'll give to the act in which an actress is sandwiched between her two costars. The principle of classic double penetration is very simple: The girl is penetrated anally and vaginally at the same time, with one guy in front and the other behind.... If you decide to put a D.P. in your film, you will learn that this kind of sex is sometimes more exciting on screen than in real life. You'll face several major difficulties: The two actors must stay hard throughout, which is no easy thing. The actor who is below is limited in his movements and often finds himself unable to thrust back and fourth. After a few minutes stagnating there, he winds up soft and naturally falls out of the actress."

— Ovidie, *Osez... tourner votre film X* (Dare... to Make an X-Rated Film)

ch 4. The Perfect Triangle

A penis in one hand, while the other hand pushes against the curved hollow of a writhing groin. An energetic and determined blond lover, and then a mild, slightly timid, dark-haired boy. Every part of me is being touched. They only take their hands away to touch me somewhere else. Fingers moving about my body, my mouth enjoying all sorts of attention.... I feel like I'm being tossed about, explored, taken care of. And then there's that ecstatic feeling of being the absolute center, the sun, the crucible. Enjoying and being enjoyed, passing the vibrations of one guy's desire to another through my skin. I am the link, the nucleus, the one and only center.

— Anna Rozen, *Plaisir d'offrir, joie de reçevoir*
(The Pleasure of Giving, the Joy of Receiving)

Having finished our study of heterosexual threesomes, let's now take a look at bisexual groupings. This is one of the most commonly depicted situations in erotic art and one of the most fantasized about in real life. A triangle of bisexual partners offers almost unlimited combinations. Each member can have sex with the others individually or simultaneously, and no inhibitions get in the way. Here, a threesome takes on its full meaning. The guys and gals have the privilege of fulfilling urges toward both sexes on the same night. Having sex with a guy and then a girl—or with both together—is an invitation you shouldn't refuse!

One Guy, Two Girls—Bisexual Variation

THE GIRLS ARE THE SHOW Guys, this is your chance to watch a real-life version of the porn you're used to seeing on television. You lie down on the bed, fall into a pile of pillows, and two women take their clothes off in front of you and begin kissing. They feel each other's breasts and finger each other's sexes, all the while showing off. You, naturally, masturbate.

Those porn films, you will discover, hide as much as they show. Porn directors construct scenes for an audience of heterosexual men. But sex between women covers a wider territory than men are thought to be interested in. In real life, you will see positions, looks, and sounds that you've never seen or heard before, and that are a joy to watch.

And this is just the first course. Even more delicious things will follow. After the women have finished coming together, they are going to play with you, and you can come with them. Isn't it wonderful?

Well, of course, it is not always that simple. Female bisexuality can't be forced, and some women definitely enjoy it more than others.

POSITIONS A threesome with two girls who are bisexual, or who at least don't mind touching each other, opens the door to all sorts of positions. In a hetero threesome, the only thing the girls can do is watch each other. Bisexual ladies can do a lot more.

69 PLUS The two girls are in a 69 position, one on top of the other or lying on their sides, enjoying mutual, passionate cunnilingus. Ari, the guy, flutters about, penetrating one girl and then the other (see Figure 4.1). As he slides into Béatrice's vagina, he feels Carla's mouth on his testicles. And when he comes around to Carla, Béatrice seizes the opportunity to kiss him. Of course, he needn't switch girls at all—he can stay with just one if everyone prefers it that way. The other will find an opportunity to enjoy him later.

If Ari is about to come, the three of them may enjoy a variation. He pulls out of Carla just before finishing, and Béatrice sucks on his penis until he comes.

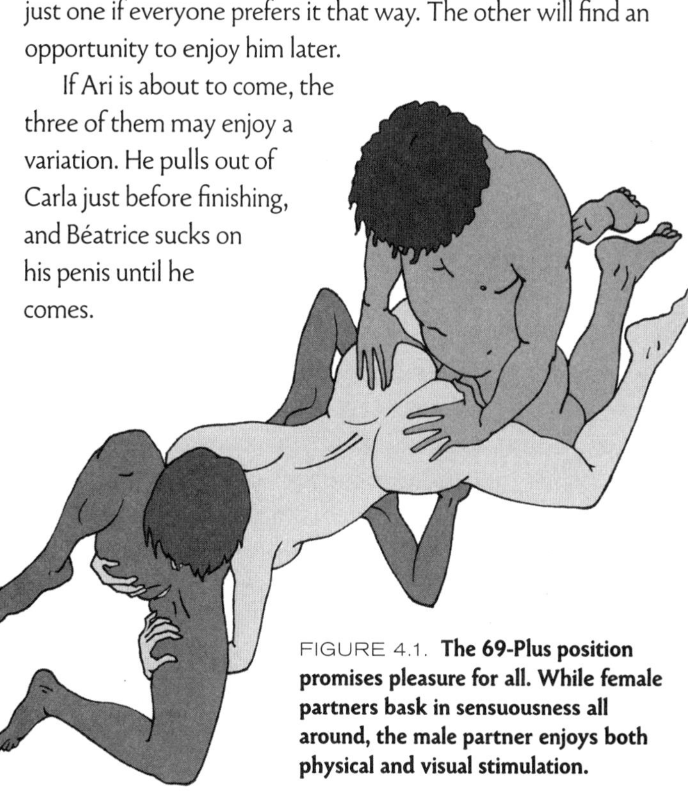

FIGURE 4.1. **The 69-Plus position promises pleasure for all. While female partners bask in sensuousness all around, the male partner enjoys both physical and visual stimulation.**

Fascination, a French magazine, recently depicted such a scene in an article by Jean-Pierre Bouyxou. They noted that it involved a "sapphic Auraristhaka combined with intercourse from behind." *Auraristhaka* is a fancy word for "cunnilingus." The engraving was originally an illustration accompanying a work by the extravagant eighteenth-century French writer Rétif de la Bretonne. The *Femme Sylphide* (Sylphic Girl) shows a couple enjoying each other in the 69 position. One girl, done up like a countess, is straddling the guy while he performs cunnilingus on her. A second girl, naked but for a headband, assists. Says *Fascination*, "The official bootlickers are here assisted by a helper of loose morals. The 69 performed in this way is an exquisite position for games involving multiple partners."

LA BOIS-LAURIER RELATES THE TALE OF HOW HER BODY RESTORED A LOVER'S EXTINGUISHED VIGOR

La Bois-Laurier is a character in the erotic novel *Thérèse Philosophe* (Thérèse the Philosopher). She tells Thérèse about a night she spent with her friend Minette and Minette's lover:

"I had to turn over on my belly, and they put about three or four pillows under me. My arse stuck high up into the air. Then they bunched my skirts, petticoat, and chemise under me so that I was absolutely naked from the navel on down. Minette lay down upon her back and her head rested between my thighs. The hairs around my cunt framed her face like a wig: Bibi undressed

> his darling Minette and laid himself down on top of her, resting upon his hands. In this position her face, my cunt, and my arse were all right in front of his nose. He licked and slurped without distinction. Now his tongue was between Minette's lips, then between my thighs, up my arsehole, into my pussy, and back between Minette's lips again. He even started to lick my buttocks. And meanwhile his member started to grow again and he began to pump away. Minette's hand guided his member back into her cunny and she began to swear and move her behind rapidly. I had turned my head around to get a good look and laughed till I ran out of breath. After they had labored for what seemed like an hour, the two lovers finally reached their climax."

LICKING THE AMAZON The guy lies down on his back, preferably on the side of a bed, his legs dangling to the floor. One of the girls sits on his lap with her back to him, skewering herself on his penis. The other girl kneels down in front of the first and begins to kiss everything that comes her way—her girl friend's clitoris, her guy's penis, his testicles, too. She can even kiss his anus or stick a finger or two inside.

THE DINER TAKEN FROM THE REAR You can guess the layout for this position. Caroline will explain how to get there—she's the heroine of the erotic nineteenth-century novel, *The School for Girls*.

> "Come, come, my friends, have a little patience. First I'm going to place myself in this armchair, one thigh here, one there. Now Marie, come here;

place yourself on your knees before me, between my legs. Take my buttocks in your hands. Good, that's it. Bend your head to my mound and let your mouth touch the lips with your tongue.... How well you understand!... Now you, Mr. Bigshot, I hope that this position is to your liking. What a perspective I've prepared for you! Now, no errors, please! I've chosen this posture as the most suitable for your attack, which shall, without too much pain, liberate this flower that Marie has kept for you. Now, each of you take up your task with passion and skill. With such a big fellow, I can vouch for success.

"(The group arranges itself and things go well at first. The tip of the vigorous Priapus, smeared with a fragrant cream, and pushed with skill, penetrates without too much difficulty and the extreme pleasure that Marie experiences from Caroline's caresses makes her forget all pain. She makes a movement that is so violent that the feared member goes in right up to the hairs. In spite of herself, a cry escapes Marie.)"

THE HORSEWOMEN A position worthy of your dreams, gentlemen—the guy is in one girl's vagina as he performs cunnilingus on the other. It is even more outrageous when the girls are bi. They can kiss and fondle each other as they both straddle the man and enjoy his attentions. The guy will welcome well-placed mirrors, even if he has to twist his neck to see the action.

He might find it easiest to lie down and use pillows to raise his torso. The girl he's going down on will kneel above his face, and if she wants to switch it up, she can also offer her breasts. The other girl will know what to do. Of course, the girls can trade places if they like.

THE MISSIONARY AND THE HORSEWOMAN One girl lies down and the second comes over to offer her sex for a little cunnilingus. Next comes the guy, who puts himself between the thighs of the first girl. He begins to penetrate her missionary style (see Figure 4.2). There are all sorts of possibilities for the next step. In one of my favorites, the guy leans forward, supporting himself with his arms on the floor or bed, and kisses the breasts of the woman who's straddling their mutual lover. You can try this position on your sides, too, with the guy and one girl lying face-to-face, as the second girl slips in between them, offering her vagina to the man and her mouth to the other girl. (Don't worry, it is easier to do than to describe.) The girl

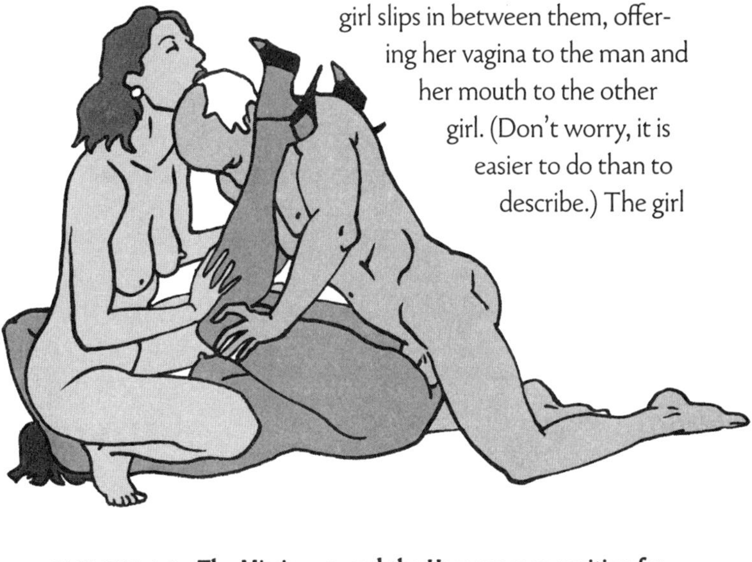

FIGURE 4.2. **The Missionary-and-the-Horsewoman position for one guy and two bisexual girls combines the strengths of two very sexually satisfying positions for explosive multiple-partner play.**

being penetrated should have no problem enjoying the situation. She can play with the genitals of the other lady while the guy has sex with her. She can also flick her tongue into the girl's vagina in sync with the guy's thrusts into her vagina.

Gamiani, or Two Nights of Excess, an erotic novel attributed to the nineteenth-century French writer Alfred de Musset, tells us about this position:

> **"The Countess was shaking like a soul possessed. Fanny's kisses had diverted her attention from my best efforts. To take my revenge, I decided to turn things around. I threw Fanny onto the Countess so that I could attack the noble lady with all my might. Suddenly, we were all mixed up and seized by pleasure."**

DOGGY-STYLE LOVE The two girls are holding each other, stroking each other, kissing, enjoying the movements of each other's fingers and tongue, nibbling on each other's nipples. One is lying on the floor enjoying these caresses, while the second one is straddling her—and offering her behind to the guy who takes her doggy-style.

INTERMINGLING LEGS One of the most satisfying sex positions for lesbians or bisexual women involves twisting their legs together and bringing their genitals face to face. In olden times, it was called *fricarelle*. As described in *Dare... to Try Kama Sutra* (which I coauthored with Axterdam):

> **"The only point of contact is the genitals. Stuck together, they guarantee mutual stimulation of erotic zones such as the clit and the labia—and of nothing else. The hands are free, and they may**

be used to caress the legs, to feel up the ankles, or to massage the feet of your friend. According to one sexologist, 'This is a sexual position that requires a deep knowledge of the other's body and a solid physical and psychological intimacy within the couple.'"

It won't take long for the girls to reach a peak. So what can a man do while this is going on? Naturally, he can get one of the girls to give him some nice fellatio.

Sylvain, another man I met on the Internet, relates this story of his first threesome, during a stay in Arras, a town in the northeast of France:

THE GIRLS OF ARRAS

"I met the girls on a café terrace at the central square. For a few minutes, I eavesdropped on their conversation. They were desperate to find a guy to keep them company on that long afternoon of Easter Monday. Neither said it out loud, but both were dying to bed someone. Yet their friends must have stopped looking at them in that way long ago, for all they seemed to do was to laugh nervously and fiddle with their cell phones. Neither pretty nor ugly, they were nice enough, and I approached them. I don't remember what I said, probably something along the lines of, 'If I were younger and more handsome than I am, I would offer myself as your devoted servant—the kind you're looking for so desperately in your phone books.'

"We talked for hours. We dropped double entendres. Occasionally our conversation turned outright risqué. Life seemed more interesting with them around, so I suggested something more intimate. 'The best place to finish our afternoon,' I said, 'would be a cozy studio with a big tub and a very big bed.'

"Béatrice, the larger and more fleshy of the girls, responded, 'That sounds just like my apartment.' A few minutes later I found myself in her studio, just beneath the rafters of an old building in Arras's center. Béatrice and Carla had never had sex with each other before, but I knew from our conversations that they sometimes bathed together nude in the North Sea around Berck-Plage. Undressing each other, we made a mess of the place. Béatrice and Carla were quickly down to their bras and panties, their excitement obvious and their cheeks ablaze. Meanwhile, they'd stripped me of my t-shirt and pants. An erection peeped through my underwear, but they pretended not to see it. The two of them were a little chubby, and their skin had that milky-white quality that's typical of girls from the north of France. But they were nonetheless pretty, and my appetite was whetted. I undid their bras and began to kiss the breasts of one while stroking those of the other. It was Béatrice who took my penis out of my underwear and began to kiss it as I went on biting and stroking Carla's breasts. We took a long bath together, in a tub too small for the three of us. As we lathered up, we chatted. I kissed one and then I kissed the other. Carla and Béatrice wanted me to judge their bodies. They kept asking me what I thought of their chests, their butts, their little pussies. Carla's thighs were a little thick and her ass was larger than what current standards of beauty deem fashionable. But her bust was magnificent, with beautiful dark nipples. Béatrice was slighter, and just a little bit plump. Her pubic hair was all in a tuft and she had little pointy breasts.

"We couldn't help but find ourselves in bed together. This was my first time having sex with two girls. Before, whenever I imagined being with two women, I always wondered how to satisfy two pussies at the same time. If I had sex with each of them, coming twice, I would make the second one wait. Instead, should I spend a couple of seconds with each and go back and forth?

"But nothing happened as expected. It all turned into a big, joyous fray. Little cries of joy were heard constantly. Two mouths fought over my penis, two girls ate each other out in an ecstatic 69, condom wrappers were opened continually, positions got strange and crazy. Béatrice lay down on her stomach. Carla lay on top of her and wrapped her arms around her friend, massaging Béatrice's breasts as I had sex with one and then the other. I only came three or four times, but each was after extraordinary, boundless love-making. We gave each other oral sex, creating a perfect triangle. I took Carla in the rear

while she kissed Béatrice's pussy. I came in Béatrice's mouth while Carla jerked her off. It was a delicious day and night, finishing only at dawn on Tuesday. Before I left, the two girls decided to give me a going-away present. They offered me their beautiful mouths one last time, and in their hands I came after one last divine and infinite moment."

A FOURTH INVITEE What if someone brought an extra participant? Not a person, but an object—a dildo. An engraving by Paul-Emile Bécat explores the possibility. It illustrates a novel by Pierre Louÿs, the *Histoire du roi Gonzalve et des douze princesses* (Story of King Gonzalve and the Twelve Princesses). The king—we know he's the king because of his crown and cape—is on his knees, while a woman, also on her knees, is fellating him and stroking his balls. A second girl is behind the first, penetrating her with a strap-on (though that's not to say that men can't enjoy this sex toy for prostate pleasuring too!). The journalist who wrote the article from the French magazine *Fascination* that I mentioned earlier in this chapter notes, "Penetration with an artificial penis is a simple embellishment that titillates a man as he performs erotic tricks with two women." Of course, in the novel, the two girls are the king's daughters, but that's another issue....

◎ One Girl, Two Guys—Bisexual Variation Combining two bisexual guys and one heterosexual girl can be a recipe for some unusual pleasures—and hot memories. Having sex with a girl is one thing; being anally penetrated by a guy at the same time is quite another. Sucking off a guy gives you one kind of sensation; having a second guy inside you at the same time gives you something different. See for yourself. You can do more than just think about it.

> **"My boyfriend and I had a MMF. We'd been wanting to for a while, and we had the luck of knowing a guy willing to experiment. So we invited him over, and we talked for a long time, even though we'd already talked about experimenting with him. The evening began quietly. We looked at pictures of the two of us, we talked about stripteases, we did a striptease. Everything went very well, and everyone enjoyed the evening. We finished with a threesome."**
>
> — Anonymous woman posting on a website for sex advice

So with the story of that positive experience as our starting point, let's look at the possibilities for a MMF threesome: male + male + female.

THE GUYS ARE THE SHOW Start the same way our informant from the message board suggests: with a striptease, a show. Anita sits comfortably on the bed, her back against a pile of pillows, and enjoys. The two men, Brian and Charles, start stripping. This is the appetizer for a hot feast that will soon follow, with kissing, stroking, sex, and more.

POSITIONS AND SITUATIONS Here's another story, this one told by Angèle, a girl I know. It is called, "The Festival of the Bearded Men." Angèle is a redhead. Having seen her naked at a swimming pool, I can tell you that she has light skin and little breasts ending in large areolas. Her tummy is slightly round, and her little pink mound can be seen by all, for she shaves off every trace of hair. Moreover, she's cute, with a fresh young face and a lively laugh. She laughs especially hard when telling this story.

> "I met them at Fury Fest, a hard rock music festival in Reims that ended suddenly because of a violent thunderstorm. They were both burly guys, with beards and tattoos, clad all in leather. I immediately thought they were of that homosexual subculture we call 'bears'—and I was partly right. But they were more than that. To help me out of the rain, they offered to take me into their van. The inside was like Versailles, Led Zeppelin style. It was full of mauve fur and lamps made to look like the heads of dead people. All in very good taste.
>
> "We chatted and waited for the rain to stop. Meanwhile, we were gulping down a case of beer, and the demon liquor got us pretty relaxed. Dick and Danny took my clothes off and started taking advantage of my breasts. Then I stripped them. I discovered Dick's Japanese tattoos and Danny's eagles. We had a threesome. It felt almost conventional. I sucked off one and then the other, and then both together, until finally my mouth began to hurt. Then Danny had sex with me while Dick rubbed his body against mine. In the back of a Dodge Caravan, suddenly turned into a bachelor pad, I had an orgasm like no other.
>
> "Then Dick and Danny said something like, 'Watch what we do,' and they began to have sex right in front of me. I was sprawled across the mauve fur, completely dumbfounded by the

show these two hairy men were giving me, as they touched and had anal sex with each other like wild animals. It was gentle and violent at the same time.

"Afterwards, Danny kneeled down in front of me while Dick penetrated him from behind. Every time Dick thrusted, I saw Danny's penis swing toward me. Soon I couldn't resist and I glided between Danny's legs and took his penis in my mouth. Dick screamed as he came, leaving me to finish Danny off. But I didn't want him to come in my mouth—that would have been a disappointment. So I turned around and offered him my ass. The noise of a condom being unfolded drove me crazy. Danny took me up the ass, and he came a few seconds later—the best seconds of my life."

DOUBLE PENETRATION This position works whether the guys are bi or straight. The bisexuals, however, may enjoy it more; they won't be scared of touching each other. In fact, that will be a bonus. They can seek out contact between the erect penises, during or after penetration. And they can touch each other before beginning, too. In fact, the woman may not mind watching as they masturbate each other before starting in on her.

FRONT AND BACK One of the guys gives head and penetrates the girl simultaneously. This must be a first-class fantasy for bisexual men. On his knees, one guy pleasures the woman doggy-style, while the other man stands in front of him, offering his penis (see Figure 4.3 on the following page). There are plenty of positions from which to try this.

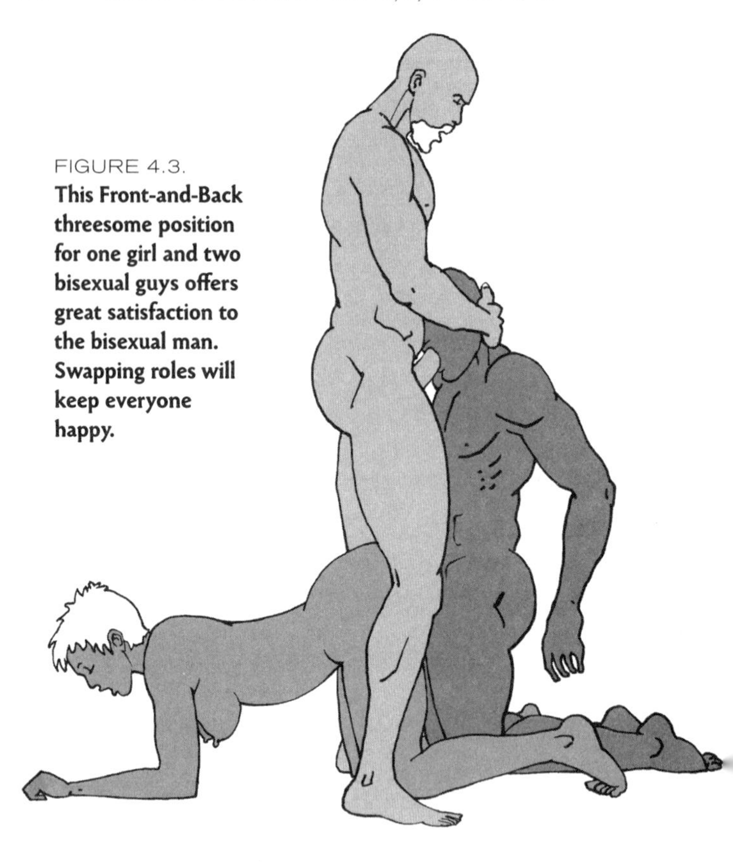

FIGURE 4.3.
This Front-and-Back threesome position for one girl and two bisexual guys offers great satisfaction to the bisexual man. Swapping roles will keep everyone happy.

THE TWO-HOSED HOOKAH The girl satisfies one guy orally while he satisfies the other guy, also orally—do you follow? Of course, the guy in the middle has the best part here and should take advantage of it. This operation works in a whole array of positions. For rest and relaxation between bouts with grander positions, I recommend that all three of you lie down on a big bed, creating a chain of your privates and your mouths. Once in a while, you'll want to switch up the links. If A is going down on B, who's going down on C at first, later on A and B can change positions, and then B and C, and so on.

THE ASSAILANT ASSAILED *L'Enfileur Enfilé* (The Assailant Assailed) is the name of a painting from 1906, probably by Paul Avril, that illustrates an underground edition of Friedrich-Karl Forberg's *Manuel d'érotologie classique* (Manual of Classic Erotology). A young woman, dressed and done up in a vaguely ancient Greek style, is lying on a sofa in an oriental room. She's lifting her legs up and resting her ankles on the shoulders of a

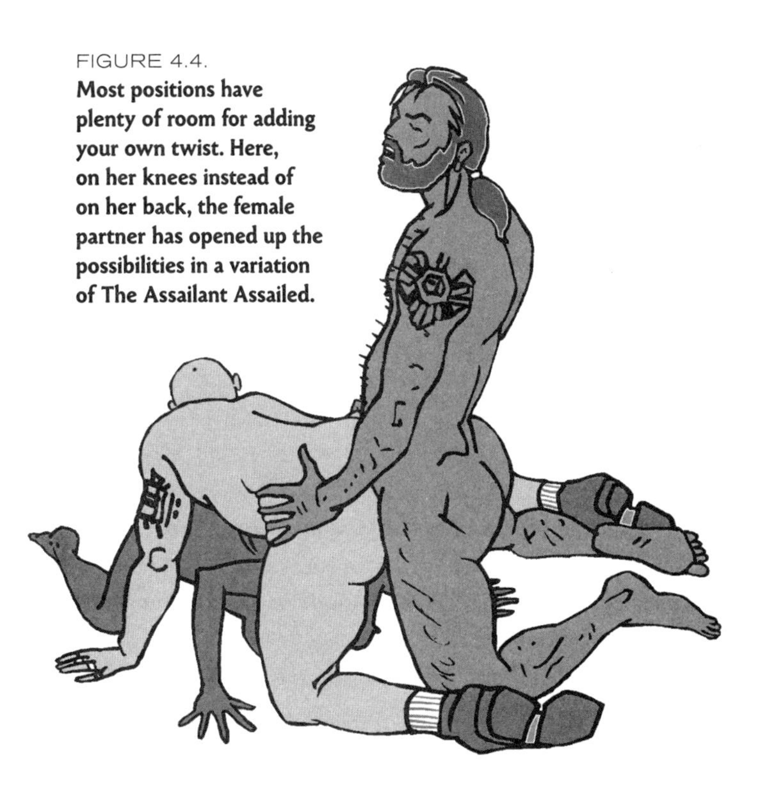

FIGURE 4.4.
Most positions have plenty of room for adding your own twist. Here, on her knees instead of on her back, the female partner has opened up the possibilities in a variation of The Assailant Assailed.

young man, also vaguely Greek (although it is difficult to tell, because he's naked). He is having anal sex with her. A second guy, with virile good looks and muscles sculpted from marble, strikes a military pose as he anally penetrates the man penetrating the woman. The writer for Fascination remarks, "In the heat of a threesome, one might well want to be ass-fucked by another man. One is screwing a woman at the same time, so one's honor is, in effect, safe" (from accusations of homosexuality).

That same edition of *Fascination* (issue 25) that we have referred to previously in this chapter shows an identical scene, also drawn by Paul Avril. A woman is lying on a sofa, a man slides himself into her, and a second man is anally penetrating the first—but here the participants are disguised as monks.

CONGA LINE "Two are penetrating and two are being penetrated—but there are only three people in all!"

This is a position made popular by the French erotic novelist Emmanuelle Arsan. One of the guys has sex with a girl as the second guy has anal sex with him. It is easy to imagine, once you understand the principle. The easiest way of putting it in place is for all three to be standing. The girl supports herself against a wall and offers her ass to the first guy, who offers his to the second (see Figure 4.5). Or you can try it lying down. That's more relaxing, even if it is harder to get started.

The girl can also lie on her back and put her legs around the neck of the guy anally penetrating her—she can then feel herself pushed around by a group of guys, which is certainly a unique sensation, although not, perhaps, an erotic one. The two men might want to trade positions halfway through. But if they do, they should remember to change condoms, too.

EMMANUELLE, FOLLOWING MARIO'S ADVICE, OFFERS HER BODY TO A SIAMESE *PAYSAN*

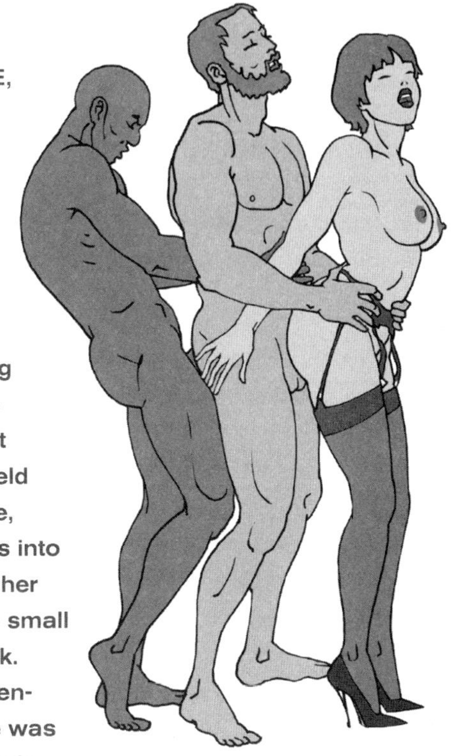

FIGURE 4.5. **Although strenuous, the Conga Line is exciting just to think about. Try it both standing and lying down.**

"She took off her skirt and [lay] down on the divan, leaning back against the enchantingly soft cushions. She held her legs out wide, pushed her heels into the rug, and slid her arms around the small of the man's back. He entered her tentatively. When he was all the way in, Mario, who had been sitting next to Emmanuelle waiting for her to be ready, stood up and put himself behind the peasant. He took hold of the man's waist and Emmanuelle felt Mario's hands touch hers.

"She heard him moaning softly out of pleasure. Sometimes, the moans came close to being screams.

> **"'Now I'm in you. I'm piercing you with a blade twice as sharp as a common man's. Do you feel it?'**
>
> **"'Yes,' she said. 'I like it.' The hard penis of the Siamese pulled out three-quarters of the way and then, unrelenting, it returned. The thrusts sped up. She didn't care whether Mario was going to let him come. She screamed, and the two men combined their screams with hers."**
>
> — Emanuelle Arsan, *Emmanuelle*

THE HORSE AND DOG One of the guys is lying down, having anal sex with the other. For his part, the friend is sitting on top with his back turned and his penis in the woman, who is on her knees in front of him. Once again, it is easier to do than to describe. As with double penetration, pleasure is not guaranteed. Everyone might find it difficult to move. But why not try it out anyway? You don't have to stay in this position all night long.

WORTH REPEATING FOR SAFETY I said it in the Introduction, but it bears repeating: "If a relation is just between two people but vaginal penetration follows anal penetration, changing condoms is crucial, for a vaginal infection can result from germs in the intestine." Obviously, this advice is even more important when a guy is penetrating the anus and vagina of two different people.

◎ **Three Girls** What if the three partners are all women?

Josée-Gabrielle Morisset, a writer and journalist, tells the story of "a threesome that was a delicacy for Monique, Françoise, and Emma" in the Canadian lesbian magazine *Corps et Âme* (Body and Soul).

"Why should we only have space in our heart for one woman? True, we can't love two women for the same reasons or in the same ways. For one thing, I had already had sexual relations with Monique, who was now living with Françoise. It all happened gradually. I made sure to be respectful of their relationship, which was very harmonious. But we liked to do things together. And we enjoyed each other."

Emma explains how they broke the ice.

"[Then,] after a late dinner washed down with drink, we were inspired to make love together for the first time. There were mouths all over the place and six hands—what do you do in bed

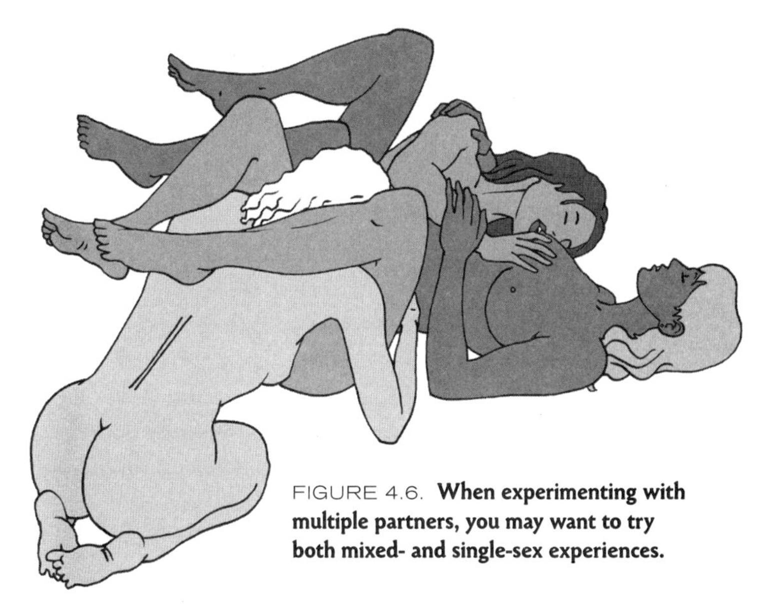

FIGURE 4.6. **When experimenting with multiple partners, you may want to try both mixed- and single-sex experiences.**

with all these parts? It's true, you lose track of whose hand, whose mouth, you're touching. You let yourself go, and it becomes very pleasant. It's also tiring—you need a lot of sexual energy. Sometimes, I have to say that Monique took positions that were weird and that didn't do much for me. But a threesome is mostly about giving yourself up, putting your feelings to the side, and thinking only about pleasure. Now that I think about it, we gave Françoise, who was a little passive, the most attention. I liked overcoming her resistances, especially since Monique and I had already been together."

She's insistent on one point: "To be harmonious, the lovers in a threesome must have a bond and a sense of humor. You always have to be ready to listen, but you can't watch yourself too closely."

The writer Charles Guillaume Étienne, describes a similar evening in his 1924 novel, *Notre-Dame de Lesbos*:

"In her place on Rue de Lille, Andréa Beuve, a blazing woman of two score years, hosts tea parties that are very much in demand. Generally ending in an orgy, everyone in attendance remains nude.... On the couches, on the rugs, on the low chairs, on the piled-up cushions, before the flickering flame of candles that cast upon women's skin a shade no other light can attain, we all go into heat.... Mouths come together, breasts fall upon stomachs, and the orgasm of one sets the desire of the others on fire."

ch 5. Two Plus Two

All four partners were thus sharing in it almost equally. The pleasure circulated: [T]hat which the duchess received from the count, she passed on to the knight, who conveyed it to Célestine, who brought it back to its initial source.

— Andréa de Nerciat, from *Félicia, ou mes fredaines* (Félicia, or My Mischief), 1772

Swapping or All Together? We call this particular sensual adventure a foursome. Let's start by considering the classic formula: two guys and two girls. It is one of the most important groupings for partner swapping, and two configurations are possible. All four partners can play together, or each person can simply swap his or her usual partner for a new one.

Swapping A foursome can simply involve an exchange of partners—and of course, macho men would like to imagine that the guys are swapping their girls. That's not to say, however, that the gals don't get off on the same type of sharing. Recent anthropological work seems to suggest this is true, but we're skeptical. Even today, sexologists tend to think of women as simple victims of their partners' desire for powerful sexuality. That's more misogynistic than partner-swapping could ever be.

Except for the pleasure to be gained by looking in mirrors, swapping in the simple sense of the word doesn't really concern us. The two couples, having exchanged the missus and the mister, typically have sex, each in their little corner. Moreover, some couples have been known to go into separate rooms with their new-found partners to consummate their friendship. Then, once they've had their fill, they join up again. Hélène Barbe, in *Osez… l'échangisme* (Dare… to Try Swinging), explains that couples in swingers clubs often have sex simultaneously, allowing fellatio, cunnilingus, and penetration to unfold at the same rhythm, so that everyone can be finished and go home at exactly the same time. This really isn't something that excites me.

Even without touching each other, two couples can inhabit the same space in a way that allows them to appreciate each other's sweaty bodies. The trick is to develop a game involving voyeurism and exhibitionism that everyone involved can enjoy. This means taking turns having sex, which is the better way to allow everyone to watch and be watched. It is the inverse of what swingers do; having sex at the same time precisely because they don't really want to see what their husband or wife is doing with someone else.

Then there are the positions where two couples have sex together, without the partners of the same sex touching each other. Remember, I'm talking about hard-core heteros here.

1691 This position and its name—1691—come from a commentator on the website www.aufeminin.com. "The two girls are in a 69 position, on their sides or one on top of the other," the commenter writes. They aren't kissing each other, however, just enjoying the show—these are heterosexual women we're talking about. "Each guy puts himself between his girl's thighs, his sex near the other lady's head. This woman can guide the guy's hands toward his partner's assets, or she can suck and touch everything that comes her way. So each girl controls what the other couple is doing, all the while enjoying the doings of another girl." (See Figure 5.1.)

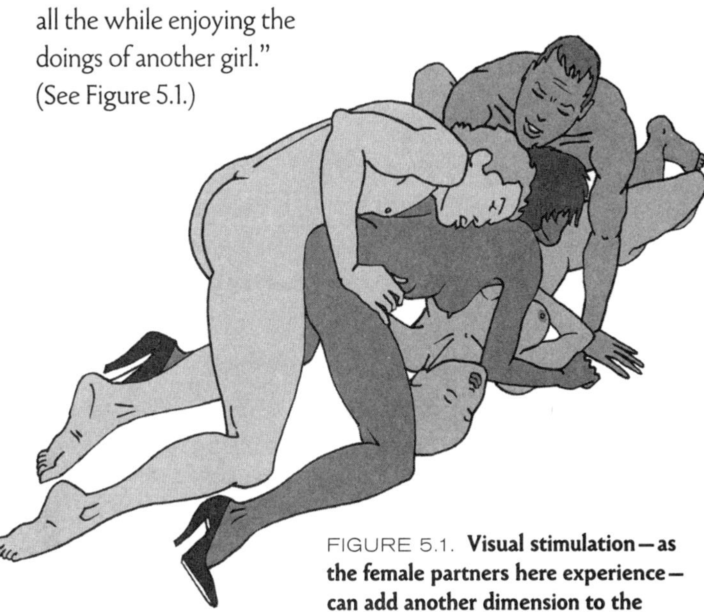

FIGURE 5.1. **Visual stimulation—as the female partners here experience—can add another dimension to the sensuousness of the 1691 position.**

HEAD TO TOE Head to toe isn't really a position; it is a situation. The two couples have sex doggy style, in such a way that they are parallel, pointing in opposite directions. This means the men are facing each other and the women are head to toe. So Ms. X is facing Mr. X as she's enjoying Mr. Y's attention.

Mr. X, meanwhile, is in Ms. Y but looking at Ms. X. Each woman can encourage her man with looks or even touches and can have fun watching what's going on between her partner's thighs.

There are plenty of other ways for two couples to have sex in the same room, of course. Catherine Millet, author of *The Sexual Life of Catherine M.*, often talks about how sex can get wanton in even the most innocent places. Two couples, under the influence of passion, can transform their house. That sofa, that couch—they'll never seem the same once you and your partner have used them to have sex with your best friends. With a little creativity, you can defile all of your furniture. You can sprawl out on the stairways or on the back lawn. The two young women can lay their torsos on an antique table, side-by-side or face-to-face, while the men enter them.

THE HOUSE IN HOLLAND

"We were meeting them in Amsterdam—a couple of friends who had been expatriates for some years. They took us to various bars and coffee-houses. Adam was courting Charlotte, my girl-friend. For my part, I remained a bit distant from Diane. Although I'd always liked her, she intimi-dated me. When we got back to Adam and Diane's place, she was the one who decreed that we had gotten hot and must all take showers. We each bathed separately, for the house had plenty of bathrooms. A little later, in pajamas and nightgowns, we met up in the living room to chat. Charlotte's gown was wide open, and Adam pre-tended to scold her for it. Making clumsy efforts

to close it, he only managed to open it further. Charlotte then gave the signal for what we were all imagining, more or less subconsciously. Instead of pushing Adam away, she pulled his face to her chest, and he began to kiss her. Immediately I felt Diane's hand gliding along the thin cotton of my Chinese pajamas, toward my penis. In an instant, I uncovered her chest. At the beach, I'd often seen her magnificent breasts, with their dark, thick nipples. Now I got to take them in my hands and kiss them as Diane took my pants off. From the corner of my eye, I noticed Charlotte's legs pointing toward the ceiling as she enjoyed Adam's vigorous thrusts. We made love together two or three times. Sometimes all four of us were in it together; sometimes we became spectators and performers. At dawn, by way of conclusion, Diana, her vagina still wet and her breasts covered with droplets of sweat, turned to me and said, 'That's what we needed.' Charlotte and I stayed in bed late that morning, having sex again and again in spite of all the energy we'd already expended on the battlefield of the night before. Together, we relived each of the moves that we'd tried with our friends. 'It's even better now,' she said, falling asleep again, as if that strange night was never to be recalled." — Benjamin

IN COUPLES OR ALL TOGETHER Some people prefer a variation on the swinger version. Instead of having intercourse with someone else's partner, everyone holds tight to his or her lover, but all four go through foreplay together. Even during sex, they keep on touching and kissing. Before everything starts, they have a summit in which they decide who is allowed to go how far. The French call this *mélangisme*, which loosely translates as "mixing it up."

I think it is even more fun to gather into a big heap. Two girls and two guys get together, ready to do anything for pleasure. They are no longer two separate couples—if ever they were—and so they're free of inhibitions about trying all sorts of positions, strokes, and kisses. In such situations, you begin to get a feeling for how vast a pleasure machine the body can be. The couples are free to be voyeurs and exhibitionists, all the more so because they don't have to worry about the effects on their long-term partners. It is no longer your husband or wife whose chest is heaving, but your other girlfriend or your other boyfriend.

◎ **All Together—Bisexual Variation** It is a great, big sensual party. Four partners, all of them bi, together in one bed. It is a scenario that all libertines dream about, and it offers so many combinations that I can't possibly explore them all. And what about when there are even more than four lovers? It gets hard to compute.

I'm going to put my cards on the table: I believe that the traditional set-up among swingers is more interesting when participants don't cringe at the idea of having sex with—or at least touching—their counterparts of the same sex. Each couple can still have sex in their own corner, but now there are four couples—or even six! Anne came to the party with Brian, and Claire arrived with David, but they can become Anne and

Claire or Brian and David. If someone wants to rest for a while, the community can turn into a threesome.

MAKE A CHAIN With fellatio and cunnilingus you can forge links that meld the four partners into a human chain. Adam is standing up, Béatrice is on all fours in front of him, sucking his penis, while Christophe lies on his back between Béatrice's legs and tastes her. Finally, Danièle goes down on Christophe. If everyone lays down, this human chain can turn into a perfect square. Each of the four bodies makes a side of a square, and everyone's face is between the legs of the guy or girl in front.

THE ROYAL COUPLE One of the guys and one of the girls are lying down, either on top of each other or side-by-side. Their hands slide across their bodies; they begin to kiss each other's lips, necks, and shoulders; and they feel each other's breasts and chests as if they were all alone. But they aren't alone. The other two members of the foursome are there, too, taking care of their partners and acting like servants or machines simply there to provide sexual gratification. They go down on the royal couple, they penetrate them—and are penetrated by them—as the royals continue with their love making. Then, of course, everyone switches roles. Since all are bi, the two guys or the two girls can become the royal couple while the other two kiss, touch, or make love to them.

THE DOUBLE LOTUS The two guys are sitting cross-legged, their backs against each other. Each woman is straddling one of the men—and having sex with him—but she can also stroke the other man, or reach over him to touch her girlfriend's face, neck, and breasts (see Figure 5.2 on the next page).

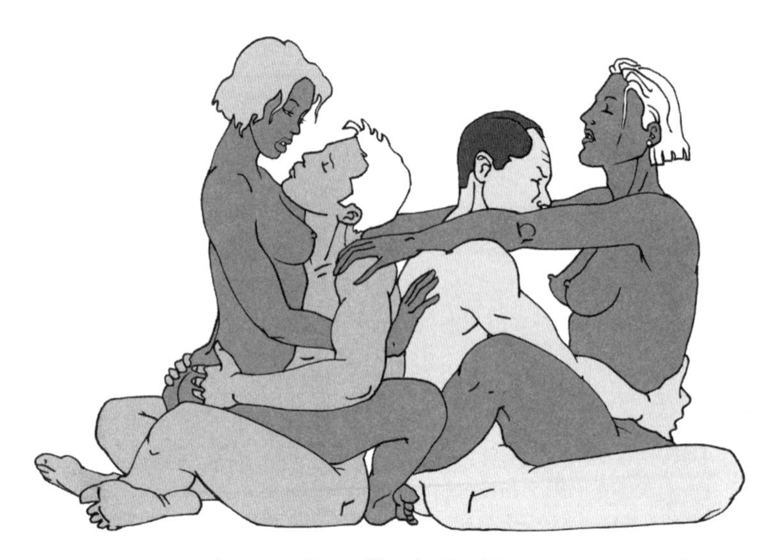

FIGURE 5.2. **Some positions, like the Double Lotus, are especially easy entry points for people just getting into multiple-partner—or multiple-couple—experiences.**

1691—BISEXUAL VARIATION I've already discussed the 1691 position. In the bisexual variant, the women in the 69 do what you would expect in a 69 position—they go down on each other and kiss each other. But this variation also allows the women to enjoy watching their men having sex with them.

ch 6. Three Against One

On my back, I could be stroked by several men while one of them, rearing up to make room and see what he was doing, would get going in my sex. I was tugged and nibbled in several places at once, one hand rubbing insistently around the available part of my pubis, another skimming broadly across my entire torso or choosing to stroke my nipples.

— Catherine Millet, *The Sexual Life of Catherine M.*

With this many people, you can do anything. Something that seems unimaginable in a "normal" sex life is likely quite doable—and done—in the unusual universe of libertinage. Take a foursome, for example. It makes for a good party. Deck your place out with soft light and cool champagne, pretty curtains and perfume. Hang mirrors all around the room so you can see everything.

◎ One Guy, Three Girls—Heterosexual Variation

One guy and three girls is an impossible task—well, almost.

For any of you macho guys who like to think of yourselves as sex machines, consider yourselves warned. You have a lot to lose in trying this. Pleasuring the three girls you've brought home is not easy, whether you pay attention to them one after the other or all at once. But even though I have said this, you don't have to give up.

The most important thing to learn is how to control ejaculation and prolong your erection. The "big" man who plans to start by coming in the vagina, anus, or mouth of all three girls isn't going to make it for very long, whereas the little guy who is miserly with his ejaculation has a better chance of keeping it up all night.

As in other situations where the girls outnumber the guys, I suggest using female condoms. This will also keep the man from having to switch condoms every time his penis goes a little limp. To begin, try some games.

THE HAREM What fantasy plays out with three girls and one guy? Naturally, the harem—but this is a harem full of demanding women. You have to build the right ambiance. Put down a Berber tent in the living room or transform it into an oriental palace. The women will be wearing gauze veils; the sultan will pretend to be angry when they come to him after the belly dance. A huge orgy will end the evening.

BLIND MAN'S BUFF This man seems lost. All naked and sweaty, he's blindfolded and looking for the three girls who are busy taking off their clothes. He has to catch them and then identify them. Don't feel sorry for him, as he's allowed to feel their breasts, their vaginas, and the rest of their bodies. In an even sexier version of this game, the guy has to guess who is kissing his penis.

THE JUDGMENT OF PARIS You are probably familiar with the following story from Greek mythology, which is also a favorite image for painters of nude women. As Marc Lemonier tells it in *Mangeuses d'hommes* (The Man-Eating Women):

"In the course of ceremonies surrounding the wedding of Thetis and Peleus, Paris was enjoined to decide who was the most ravishing of Mount Olympus's three beauties: Athena, Hera, or Aphrodite. He was supposed to give the most beautiful a golden apple on which were written the words, 'for the most beautiful one.' "

In this game, the three girls present themselves in the nude to be judged. The winner will have sex immediately with her judge, while the other two, boosted by their numerical superiority and enraged by the verdict, take part in the romp, demanding a piece of the pleasure.

A FOURSOME AMONG NUDISTS

"Our foursome began as a tennis game. Every summer since I was seven, I've gone with my family to the same nudist resort, where I meet my friends Bibi and Annie. We've gotten a lot older since we started going. Our families, who are all nudists, still think of us as 'the little ones,' but they're the only ones who do. In the last year or two, the three of us have stopped staying in our families' bungalows and instead set up a big igloo tent in the middle of the camping area. We spend our time flirting in the nude. That [first] year, Bibi, who's petite and curvy, had brought a guy or two back to the tent. While we tanned, Annie met a boy and spent her days with him until he left the camp. I, too, had sex once or twice with a sort of regular lover who often came down for vacation.

"And then one day, we played a game of tennis with Dirk, a blond and friendly Dutch guy. He completed our team for a doubles match. After we'd played, we hit the showers, which are communal and unisex. Dirk hadn't played great, and we began to make fun of him. We fondled his stomach and accused him of having a potbelly. We felt his muscles and pretended to find them too weak. Annie, who notices everything, told us later that he was already making desperate efforts not to get hard. Then we went back to our tent to drink a bottle of rosé as the night fell. Still naked, we sat down in the middle of the igloo to chat.

"I'm not sure how everything got started. Annie probably teased Dirk by kissing him on the neck or massaging his shoulder. But I still remember Bibi saying, 'I see that we're making a good impression on you.' Dirk was erect—now there was no hiding it—and he didn't seem embarrassed. He kissed each of us for a long time, one after the other, while his hands felt our breasts—Bibi's sumptuous chest; Annie's little, hard nipples; and mine, dark and large. We soon felt as if Dirk had ten hands and twenty mouths. Our hearts were on fire. I think Annie was the first to go down on him, as he slid his fingers into my pussy. It seems to me that Bibi straddled him as he rubbed our wet sexes.

"Later, much later, we made a count of what happened. Annie maintains that Dirk came in her mouth at the end of the night after having had sex with her twice. I'm sure that he also made me come twice, which was once more than I'd ever come before. Bibi claims that Dirk had anal sex with her and came on her breasts after having explored everything one can explore of her body. In vain we counted again and again, because we doubted our accuracy. Either some of us are exaggerating or he was a stallion.

"Anyway, what I remember most of all about that night is a boy with his face stuck between my breasts and whose hands no longer knew whose ass they were feeling up. We were happy, drunk on our own pleasure and the pleasure of this guy, who must have had one of the best nights of his life. Although maybe not the best, because after that, I kept him for myself and gave him plenty of other nights with lots of other kinds of satisfaction." — Claire

A LITTLE BIT OF HELP Take a count. There is one penis and three vaginas. Let's be honest: It would be hard for any man to keep them all satisfied at once. But there might be a solution. Consider taking out that dildo. Vibrating or not, made of plastic or glass, it will add something to the situation. One girl can use her expertise with it to pleasure another, as they both sit around, rudely abandoned by their man, who is enjoying the third partner. It is a typical image from porn films.

The dildo will be most effective if preparations are made for its entry. A spot of lube will do the trick, although the best lubricant is still the natural one—your fingers and your tongue preparing the way for the little gift. Using a dildo allows for its own set of variations. And who knows, you might even wind up using it on the man.

SAFER SEX TIP

When penetrating several partners in succession—even using a dildo—you will want to change condoms after each one so that vaginal or anal secretions don't get mixed together and HIV or other infections are not transmitted. This is a good idea even when moving from one orifice to another on the same partner. You want to avoid transmitting liquids from one entryway to another.

◎ **One Guy, Three Girls—Bisexual Variation** With three bisexual girls, you can explore all sorts of possibilities. Their bisexuality should be a relief to the guy, who no longer has to feel responsible for everyone's pleasure. (Foursomes are hard on him—three women can seem like twenty!)

In my experience, though, finding a foursome made up of one man and three women is a very rare combo. Mostly, it occurs in fantasies and porn, so if you can gather the right people, you are in for a truly unique experience. Positions that are only possible with this quarter meld heterosexual and lesbian love making (see Figure 6.1). And the gatherings are beautiful to look at. Having sex two-by-two or all together, the partners won't know where to put their mouths next.

ACROBATIC POSITION FROM INDIA In his book *La sexualité féminine* (Female Sexuality) sexologist Yves Ferroul explains that:

"Indian temples depict couples in acrobatic positions, flanked by two young women who help them remain in position by lifting an arm or leg, or by providing the woman with a neck to hang on to for balance. Sometimes, the man seems to misplace his hands on the thighs of his two helpers, who apparently appreciate the payoff for their participation."

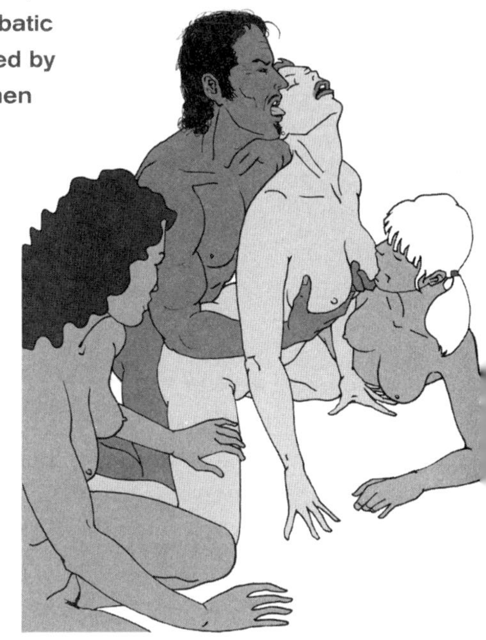

FIGURE 6.1. **Experiences involving one man and three bisexual women take the pressure off the male partner, allowing him to truly let himself go.**

The young woman being held can similarly feel up her carriers. She can even kiss them or slide a finger or two inside them, all in good fun.

SPOILED One of the girls has sex with the guy, perhaps straddling him as he's sitting cross-legged. She's the guest of honor—her two friends massage her, nibble at her breasts, indulge her anus with a finger, and kiss the nape of her neck and her earlobe (an oft-neglected sweet spot). If she wants to be nice, she can kiss them back.

One Girl, Three Guys—Heterosexual Variation

If you enjoy feeling like your body is filled up, Madam, this one's for you. Surrounded by men, you can slide one of them into each of your body's entrances. The men, meanwhile, should be attentive. There may be more of them, but that doesn't mean they should pay attention to their pleasure alone.

SHOULD YOU REALLY TRY IT? No psychologist or sexologist will suggest this to a client, nor will a boyfriend bring this up to his girlfriend. It is an extreme situation. Most readers, I suspect, will come to this section for fun stories but not for practical advice.

On the other hand, this kind of foursome is common in swingers clubs. Is this enough of a reason to try it? It is up to you. One thing is sure, though: You can always say "No," and it doesn't matter how far along you are. Anna Rozen depicts this well in *Plaisir d'offrir, joie de reçevoir* (The Pleasure of Giving, the Joy of Receiving).

> "Suddenly my partner asks me whether I want 'something else,' whether I want 'more.' My answer comes as a sigh. 'Yes, yes,' I let out, without understanding what a guy so talented could offer that would be better. 'Yes, yes,' I say, and I mean, 'anything you want, just as long as it continues.' My partner waves his free arm in a long motion, a gesture you would expect from John Wayne. But I don't pay attention. I let myself be gently

rocked by the bouncing of the carriage, without seeing the oncoming attack.

"When the two fat oafs appear, my clitoris goes soft immediately, and I throw myself at the foot of the bed, at my clothes. I yell something like 'absolutely not' as I get dressed. I'm completely sober now, my mind lucid, and I'm angry. The two guys stand there dumb and disappointed, their arms dangling down.

"My beau is the one who throws me out, in a fit of insults. 'Who do you think you are? Have you looked in a mirror recently? Get out of here, you fat pig! Get out!'

"No matter how rude it may be, there are days when saying 'No' is the right thing to do. Never allow an ambush."

CONFIDENTIAL TO WOMEN What kind of woman might try this? You???

The feminist lawyer Marcela Iacub, author of *Le Crime était presque sexuel* (The Crime Was Almost Sexual) and *Qu'avez-vous fait de la libération sexuelle* (What Have You Done with Sexual Liberation) declares:

"Instead of being a time when there is a struggle for the equality of the sexes, and especially for women to have as liberated, open, and free a relationship to sexuality as men do, the present moment sees efforts to limit male sexuality to the forms usually taken by female sexuality.... Today, we can no longer...imagine that a woman might want to be taken by ten or fifteen men. In

> **her book, Catherine Millet voices a kind of protest against this tendency. She is at once a woman who affirms her sexuality, who isn't interested in love or affection, and who takes charge of her sexuality without an axe to grind...."**

Does that describe you? Not only wanting a lot but wanting the best—and being at the forefront of a new sexual revolution? Isabelle Alonso, vice president of the French feminist organization *Chiennes de Garde* (Watch-Bitches), made a similar observation:

> **"We're imbued with a specific moral order: Supposed sexual liberation actually represents the freedom of men to use women's bodies. Women's sexuality is still muzzled. Women must still confront a system of double values that glorifies men and scorns women (a man who has sex = Don Juan; a woman who has sex = slut)."**

As you can see, if you engage in some of the foursomes presented here, you're well outside of the norms. And to highlight the double standard, note that I didn't have to have this discussion when a man found himself in the midst of three women. Still, it is your choice.

So, after taking all the precautions you feel necessary, lead your three pretty guys by their dicks and find a discreet place to use. It should be secluded enough that you and your male harem won't have to explain yourselves to the whole world.

CHIPPENDALES Have you never had a bachelorette party? Even if you're not about to marry the three men you've taken home, now is a good time to get a little taste of the fun. Have your lovers do a striptease for you. Consider it a little test in which they prove themselves worthy of your body by giving you a show to remember. You sit down comfortably, your hand on your cooch, and wait. Not only will the guys have to strip, but they'll have to be sexy about it. They should come and rub themselves against your body, letting you feel around in their underpants before they take them off and throw them at you.

SIX-HANDED MASSAGE Do you know everything about your body? Does it have some pleasure spots that you still haven't discovered—or, more importantly, that your lovers haven't yet found? Maybe it does.

Listen to the advice of my good friend Italo Baccardi, who wrote a *Dare...* guide devoted to helping you prepare your body for love:

> "Ignorance is often the principal obstacle to a full sexual experience. Men are often ignorant of the best ways to please women, and vice versa. Many men touch ladies as they themselves would like to be touched—as if the woman were a man. They think about pleasuring her in reference to their own pleasure. This discrepancy is clear when men and women are interviewed separately about women's erogenous zones (see a study that appeared in *20 Ans* [20 Years Old]). While women identified twelve areas that they enjoy having touched in the heat of the moment, men only knew, on average, about four. So you can see, dialogue within the couple is important and incomplete. If you, sir, know only four of a

woman's erogenous zones, I won't leave you in the dark. The twelve are: the breasts, the earlobe, the small of the back, the armpits, the navel, the behind, the clitoris, the vagina, the inside of the thighs, the back of the knee, and the feet."

One man can't take care of all of these zones at once. But with three men, it is easy—and each is responsible for only four areas (see Figure 6.2).

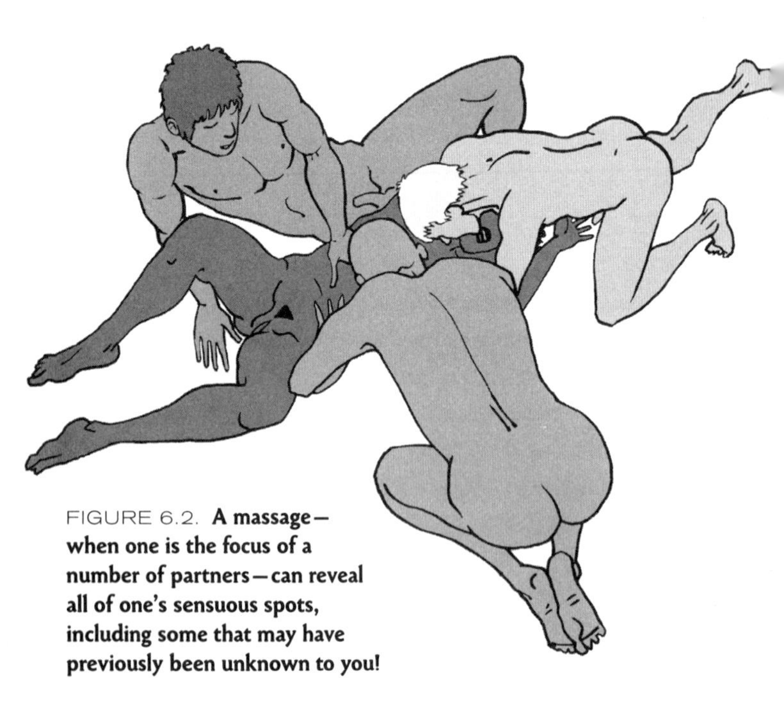

FIGURE 6.2. **A massage—when one is the focus of a number of partners—can reveal all of one's sensuous spots, including some that may have previously been unknown to you!**

To finish the massage, a guy can slide between the girl's legs and put his mouth to her sex while the other two play with her breasts, one each.

POSITIONS AND SITUATIONS Being surrounded by men should never be uncomfortable for the woman. If she chooses well, her lovers will cuddle with her, pamper her, and, above all, they'll make her forget the dangers she might feel in their numbers. Which isn't to say they won't take her like wild animals, too. Now, how to work this delightful band of sex fiends into pleasurable positions?

THE BOAT The woman straddles one of the men and masturbates the other two, each of whom is on his knees (see Figure 6.3). It is as if she were paddling a rowboat. Despite what pornography might make you think, the movements don't have

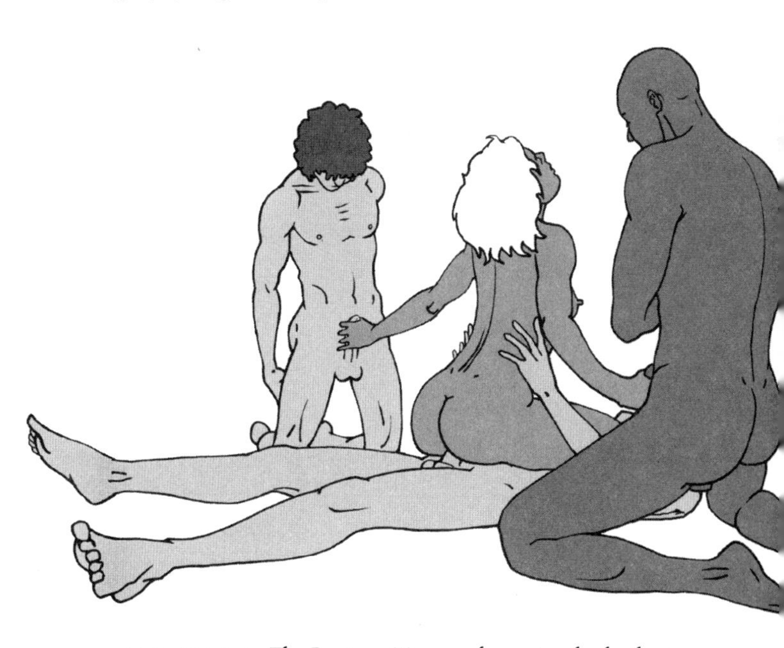

FIGURE 6.3. **The Boat position can be curiously rhythmic and deeply arousing for all, even in its simplicity.**

to be frantic. Porn films are unable to illustrate the gentleness of sex—this is especially true of films that show a foursome.

PULLING A TRAIN This is one of the most common fantasies that makes a girl want to try having sex with three guys. She gives herself to her lovers without pause or end. She offers her body to these anonymous penises and enjoys as they thrust, come in her, pull out, and are immediately replaced. Three men, all of them in a state of furious excitement, can keep you moaning and groaning for what will seem like hours—by the time the third has finished, the first will certainly be ready again. You'll feel as if you're not having sex with three guys, but with five, six, or more. Ideally, each new penis will raise your excitement to a new level.

For this to work, the girl has to be comfortable. She's going to be in the same position for a long time. She might bend over on a mattress, allowing her torso to fall over a cushion and her behind to lift up into the air for the men. All she need do is hold on to the cushions as she comes. Or she can lie on her back, offering her body in a traditional missionary position.

Pulling a train is often a submissive fantasy, and the anonymity of the men is a plus. If that's the woman's wish, she has a couple of options to help keep the guys anonymous. The simplest is a blindfold. Alternatively, the room can be totally darkened so everyone is anonymous—just a group of wet, hard sexes.

But women and men can get off on things other than submission and anonymity. The best thing about pulling a train is that the girl is kept satisfied. To help, she should actively help her lovers get hard again after they are exhausted. She can kiss and handle their manhoods while another honors her with his.

THE SWING Having this many men around can be practical. The woman can turn them into furniture. Two men hold her in their arms while a third has sex with her (see Figure 6.4). One more fantasy comes true. Plus, furniture with a mouth to kiss doesn't appear every day. Yet that's what she gets when she orders two of her lovers to support her. They can be standing or on their knees as they hold her, but she'll want to hold tight either way.

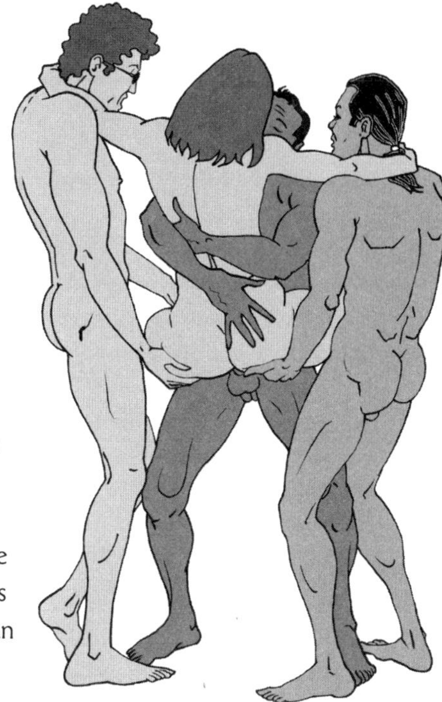

FIGURE 6.4. **Some positions, like The Swing, can't help but fulfill fantasies even as they satisfy partners.**

ARE YOU POLYITEROPHILIC?

If being with this many guys or girls barely gets you excited, you might be a polyiterophile. What does that mean? Let's see what the dictionaries say. Those with polyiterophilia (from the Greek *polus*, many; the Latin *iteratirus*, multiple times; and the Greek *philia*, love of) can't reach orgasm until they've had sex with many partners.

> **According to John Money, author of *Love and Love Sickness*, "Its definitive characteristic is that a man or woman builds up his or her responsiveness towards orgasm alone or with a partner by reiterating the same activity many times with many different partners in a limited period of time. The activity varies but it is usually some form of manual, oral, anal, vaginal, or penile manipulation. To illustrate, a homosexual male with the syndrome of polyiterophilic fellatio will be able to reach an orgasm with his partner only after accumulating a dozen 'blow jobs,' that is, acts of fellatio, on different men at, say, a steam bath or sauna club."**

TRIPLE PENETRATION

This might be as extreme as it gets. The question is, dear lady: Are you sure to get off from it? That will depend on the strength of your desire and excitement. I must admit that it is difficult to move when you have some guy's penis in the mouth, a second in the anus, and a third wandering around your vagina.

There's no ideal position for triple penetration, although the most common, popularized in pornographic images and films, is easy to imagine (see Figure 6.5). Adam lies down on his back, Béatrice sits down facing him and puts his penis in her vagina, and Charles comes behind her and has anal sex with her, while Dénis, on his knees next to the other three, offers his erect penis to Béatrice's lips. For her part, she risks leaving the party a little stiff.

This is another one of those positions that figures in porn films but is neither as exciting nor as comfortable in real life. In fact, the most pleasure might come from the excitement of breaking a taboo and fulfilling a fantasy.

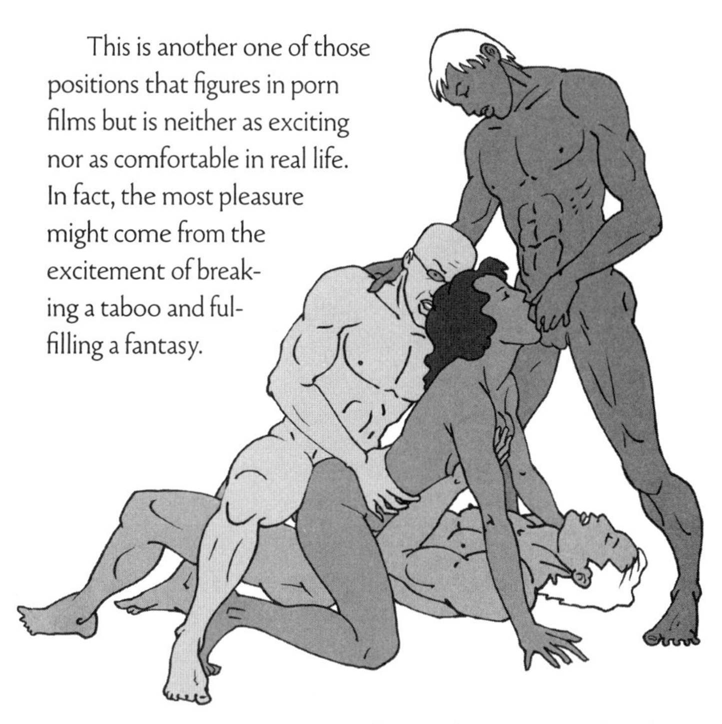

FIGURE 6.5. **Some positions, such as Triple Penetration, though exciting, can be physically demanding on one or more of the partners—a fact that all partners should recognize from the start.**

SPERM SHOWER In an X-rated film, after a girl has sex with several men, they invariably ejaculate on her body. This should be relegated to porn films. Legend has it that the practice, *bukkake*, originated in Japan as a punishment for unfaithful women. Once discovered, these women were tied up in the town square while all the men of the town ejaculated on them. Moreover, the smell of large quantities of sperm has sent more than one porn star reaching for a bucket to vomit in. So my advice: Avoid it completely!

One Girl, Three Guys—Bisexual Variation If the three guys in the foursome are all bisexual, the girl is likely to find herself at a party consisting of mustachioed fellators and virile sodomites. Let's hope she finds this sexy—especially since the three hoodlums will probably know how to satisfy her, too. In these situations, where anyone is liable to have sex with anyone else, people begin to look like an Erector Set—the pieces can be put together in all sorts of different ways, and still create something spectacular.

MAKE A CHAIN (ENCORE) Adrien, Brian, Claire, and David are trying out a new game: a human chain. The rule is simple: Each of the four partners must be either giving or receiving pleasure at any moment, or both, and the four players all have to be knotted together. The links, of course, will be penises, vaginas, anuses, and mouths. Adrien is on his knees, his hard penis being sucked by Brian, who is on all fours. Claire has her face between Brian's legs and is fellating him. David is lying between Claire's legs, supporting himself on Brian's back while having sex with Claire.

You got it? You need another example? This one follows the same principle, but Claire begins the chain. She lies on her back, spreading her legs out wide and upward. Adrien, who is on all fours between her thighs, goes down on her while Brian, lying on the floor with his head between Adrien's thighs, sucks Adrien off. At the same time, David has anal sex with Brian.

Or there's a third possibility: Adrien is standing, his sex in Claire's mouth. She's on her knees while Brian, lying on the floor, has slid between her legs and is giving her cunnilingus. David is sitting on Brian's penis. All four are moving slowly and harmoniously.

One last arrangement? The four musketeers are all standing. Adrien has anal sex with Brian who is being sucked off by Claire, while David penetrates her as he stands firmly behind her.

We could go on.... The idea is simple, and the situations are nearly infinite in number and character. Is it as fun to experience as it is to describe? You'll find out. But there's certainly a crazy element in these positions—a need for athleticism and aesthetics—that will attract those who enjoy unique moments. The one downside: It is extremely difficult to get everyone to orgasm at the same time. But that shouldn't keep you from trying. At the very least, everyone will have had fun.

A PEEK INTO A PARISIAN SAUNA

Ariane is forty years old. Her body doesn't fulfill the conventional standards for beauty. She is practically a giant, but anyone who has seen her having sex can tell you that this doesn't keep her from being active. Much of her sex life is thanks to her husband's bisexuality. We met them in the main room of a sauna. She was presiding over three men, one of whom had slid between her legs and was sucking her off. Next to her, Ariane's husband was doing the same to a fourth guy. The whole afternoon through, Ariane enjoyed the kisses and touches of three men, who took turns pleasuring her. When she was done with one, another would come immediately. But only mouths and hands were allowed to touch her. At the afternoon's end, her husband came over, and he was the first to have full-on sex with her, coming inside her and ending this long, exquisite moment.

ch 7. ... or More

I was meant to be with five or six
In a pinch maybe even seven
That's just who I am,
Not made for coupled love.
Why do they say that two's enough
It isn't, not for me.
If we could be with five or six
Everything would be so simple.
If we could be with five or six
Everything would be so natural.

— Serge Gainsbourg, translated from the song
"*J'etais fait pour les sympathies*" (I Was Made for Sympathies)

There's no limit. I've stopped at four partners, because I have to stop somewhere. But far larger groups get together to have sex in swingers clubs, at people's houses, and in the great outdoors. "Group sexuality," to use a term largely abandoned today, has become commodified, even as it remains taboo—a development that the prophets of the sexual revolution no doubt never expected.

Swingers Clubs What happens there?

In *Osez... l'échangisme* (Dare... to Try Swinging), Hélène Barbe gives us some idea:

"Swingers clubs are playpens for people looking for immediate satisfaction. Whether they play music or feature saunas and whirlpools, they offer private areas done up for comfortable sex. These cute areas have at least a mattress and some decoration, and some rooms go as far as to offer a place to try out common fantasies—doctor's exam tables, prison cells, or massage rooms."

There you go. A swingers club is a place to meet strangers for sex without being overly risky.

Swingers clubs are visited by singles and couples from all social groups and of all ages (over twenty-one, of course), although forty-somethings tend to predominate. The ambiance of the clubs varies in quality. Some are a little kitsch and make us laugh. The décor is silly and people's outfits are cliché. Agnès Giard, a journalist, described the worst of these clubs in her blog "Les 400 Culs" (The 400 Asses), "Promiscuity, out-of-style dancing, a shabby clientele: These clubs often seem to be stuck in the eighties. But once in a while you can have a good time."

So how do you have a good time? The only rule is to respect others—never go after the object(s) of your desire without getting confirmation of his, her, or their interest beforehand. This principle is easier to follow in clubs that allow only couples or are very selective when it comes to single men. Unfortunately, for reasons that are probably financial, more and more clubs waive their usual large entry fees for single men. In the afternoon—when they tend to come out—the presence of these men can be a real blight, and only women who are fans of gang bangs will go anywhere near the clubs.

But swingers clubs have one great virtue—they allow you to try what you would never even think of doing in your regular life. In the sanctuary of clubs, it is relatively safe to have sex with people you don't know—safer, in any case, than trying it at your place or theirs. As Daniel Welzer-Lang, sociologist and author of *La planète échangiste* (Swingers Planet), notes, swingers clubs stake their reputations largely on safety. A club can't allow undesirables or incidents. They have to take steps to guarantee the safety of women who come. I've even seen a guy ejected for no other reason than simply making a coarse gesture at a young woman, who complained about it.

◎ **An Evening in Private** Organizing an evening at home has a number of hazards. The question of who to invite is often the most difficult. Several organizers of "semiprivate" evenings, modeled on evenings of "ladies and champagne," told me that they work by slowly widening their libertine circle. An article by Gérard Lefort in the French publication *Libération* rightly emphasizes the importance of having an odd number of participants. Four people usually break up into two couples; whereas eight people tend toward four groupings. To help everyone connect, experience suggests that an odd number works best (see Figure 7.1). Go back to the chapters on trios as you think about this.

A PRIVATE EVENING WITNESSED BY MICHAEL BIERMANN

"There came this Saturday to Léonore's place several visitors: Katheline, who still hasn't heard anything from her traveler; Émile, who we'll get to

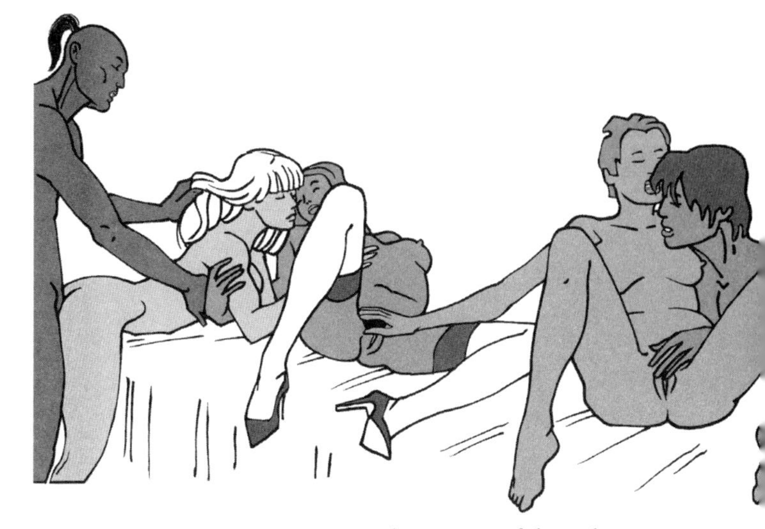

FIGURE 7.1. **Even an orgy has some guidelines that, when followed, will make it more pleasurable for all.**

know better tomorrow; Deidre, in a see-through shirt; Feyssal, with his magic dick; and, of course, Antoine. Everything was ready. Quickly, each person took his place. Ten tableaux serve to summarize the action. The author of this piece, wishing to impart to his reader the most precise descriptions possible, hereby invites the gentle reader to draw them out, if he is skilled, or have a friend draw them. In doing so he will gain a better idea of the day's shape.

"Katheline is a plump redhead, Deidre a pretty, rascally brunette, and Léonore is svelte, with auburn hair. Émile is a native of Marseille, a little stocky, while Feyssal is a handsome Berber with fine curls in his hair and Antoine is well-built though not heavy. Decorate the scene as you see fit, with pillows, fruits, bottles, and other things. Don't forget that the windows are open and the sun is streaming into the place. Now, pick up your pencils, without shame.

"First scene: Katheline kisses Feyssal, who jerks off Deidre, who goes down on Léonore. Emile rims the asshole of Antoine, who whacks off Léonore, who herself jerks off Émile."

"Second scene: Katheline sucks off Feyssal, who rims Antoine, who penetrates Katheline's ass with a dildo. Emile makes out with Deidre, who uses a dildo on Léonore, who sticks a finger up the butt of Emile."

"Third scene: Katheline is ass-fucked by Feyssal, who is making out with Léonore, who is herself getting rimmed by Katheline. Émile is fucking Deidre, who is kissing Antoine, who is being sucked off by Émile.

"Fourth scene: Katheline is ass-fucked by Feyssal, who is kissed by Léonore, who herself is being rimmed by Katheline. Émile screws Deidre, who kisses Antoine, who is being sucked off by Émile."

— Michael Biermann, *Les trente jours de Marseille* (Thirty Days of Marseille)

The scene should be set up to have an ambiance as appealing as the most tasteful clubs. I asked Amandine and Bernard for advice. These two swingers recently redecorated their bedroom to suit their erotic purposes. "The most difficult thing," Bernard says, smiling, "is to make sure that your sex palace is unnoticed by visitors—like my mother-in-law—who you don't want to let in on your private life." He takes out his blueprint, sketched on graph paper. "Everything can be moved around," he explains.

It only takes a few minutes to transform Bernard and Amandine's big bed into Bernard's idea of a sex palace. With a single tug, two drapes come down on either side of the bed, while the doors of an armoire slide open to reveal two large mirrors reflecting everything that goes on in bed. A DVD player and widescreen TV allow the couple to watch X-rated movies. The TV and DVD player are on wheels, so they can also be rolled in front of the bed. Of course the ceiling lights can be dimmed, and a kind of secret cabinet is hidden in the head of the bed. Inside, Amandine keeps her pink vibrator, lubricating jelly, a lot of colored condoms, and some scarves that she and Bernard both enjoy to attach each other and their friends to the poles of the beds.

On the evenings when action is to take place, Bernard and Amandine usually cover their bedspread with a plastic sheet, similar to those that swingers clubs put on their couches. Sometimes, Amandine goes for a finer cloth, in pink satin. It depends on the mood they want to set.

They've also decorated other rooms in the house. Bernard got some mirrors for the living room—stand-alone, so that a few minutes are enough to take them down to the cellar. At an antique store, he bought a prie-dieu (a prayer desk, with a place to kneel), which stands in a corner. Amandine likes to sit on it while offering her ass to be taken. Mother thinks it is simply decorative. A pillar made of knobby wood that stands at the foot of the stairs quickly became a favorite of Amandine's. "I love it," she says. "We turn the lights off, light some candles, and we use scarves to tie the prettiest of our invitees to the post, his hands behind his back. It's as if we had our own dungeon in the house."

In an apartment well-constructed for orgies, you should be able to wash up often and lie down wherever you like. The lights should be dimmed, and decorations should be tailored to the circumstances. Pictures of your kids and fragile ornaments should be put in the closets. Condoms should be available in various places throughout the house, and no one should be drunk, bitter, jealous, or frustrated.

ADVICE FOR SWINGERS IN PARIS

> **"Be quiet. If you see celebrities, don't harass them by asking them to tattoo their autograph on your ass. Keep your opinions of the décor to yourself, too, even if the wallpaper really is awful and you would have put the coffee table elsewhere. Finally, if you're in Paris, check out the television listings, for it's not impossible that Frédéric Taddeï has come to film the debauchery."**
>
> — Gérard Lefort, *Libération*, August 1, 2005

As for Frédéric Taddeï, the host of *Paris dernière*, a guide to the city's salacious nightlife, he reports this dialogue with a couple engaging in a night of orgies:

Taddeï: "Whose house are you in?"
A guy: "Gisèle's!"
A girl: "No, we're at Josiane's!"
The guy: "Oh, sorry. I thought you asked 'Whose ass are you in?'"

Gang Bang The gang bang, popularized by porn films, involves a woman performing a variety of sexual acts (fellatio, masturbation, various penetrations) with as many men as possible. It is a fairly rare and extreme situation. But I have seen girls enjoying and consenting to it—even without being paid—in private and in swingers clubs. Usually women seeking this type of situation come to a club alone, in the afternoon, and put themselves in the hands of a lot of men, never fewer than four or five. They lay down the rules. One woman I saw, tall and naked with brown hair, gave a lesson to a dozen guys with erections as they were about to begin stroking her breasts one afternoon. "I make the decisions, and I choose what I want. I give head but I won't swallow, and I don't kiss. Oh, and I forgot. I also like to talk." Everyone obeyed.

I don't claim to understand the sexual desires of these young women, which many sexologists refuse to admit exist. But I've always found them to be happy and determined to get what they want. They don't come with men whose fantasy they are fulfilling or who are trying to punish them. Rather, when I have seen them come with a boyfriend, he seems to be enduring the action rather than presiding over it.

So it remains a mystery.

The one person who has given any well-documented explanation at all is Catherine Millet, even if she pretended not to know the term "gang bang" when her book came out. Here's what she has to say about the extravagant pleasures in which she took part:

> **"The Porte de Saint-Cloud parking lot borders on the boulevard Périphérique and in places is separated from it only by an openwork wall. All**

I had on were my shoes, having slipped off my raincoat, whose lining iced my skin, before getting out of the car. At first, as I have said, they rammed me up against a perpendicular wall. Éric saw me 'pinned up by their pricks, like a butterfly.' Two men held me up under the arms and legs, while the others took it in turn hammering against the pelvis to which my whole person had been reduced. In these dicey situations, where there are many of them, men often fuck quickly and forcefully. I could feel the rugged shoulders of the breezeblocks digging into my shoulders and my hips. Even though it was late, there was still some traffic. The thrumming of the cars, so close they seemed to almost brush past us, lulled me into the same daze I feel at airports. With my body both freed of all weight and curled up on itself, I retreated within myself. From time to time I would glimpse through my half-closed eyes the headlights of a car as they swept over my face."

Well, there's no accounting for taste.

ch 8. Conversation Pieces

"Erotic literature that encourages men and women to have multiple partners only prepares the way for measures that we will eventually have to adopt. Compulsory polygamy, for example—and rest assured that I'm not opposed to polyandry."
— Boris Vian, French writer, poet, musician,
from *Écrits pornographiques* (Pornographic Writings)

Naked beneath the sheets, nearly asleep after an unforgettable night, you really need to rest, but you're not ready to sleep. And you're wondering whether your sexual forays are normal. This is the time to go rummaging through your DVD collection or your library. Here are some "conversation pieces," to use Gala Fur's expression from *Osez... tout savoir sur le SM* (Dare... to Learn Everything about S&M). Besides keeping you up at night, these works will keep you from growing bored between bouts.

◎ **Books for Your Night Table** Hundreds of erotic novels depict threesomes and other scenes with multiple partners. The books I cite here don't even begin to cover the matter, and you might want to look elsewhere for more erotic literature.

NOVELS

- de Musset, Alfred. *Gamiani, or Two Nights of Excess.* New York: Olympia Press, 2007.
  De Musset offers great descriptions of frenzied threesomes. It's what you would expect from a classic of erotic literature.

- Houellebecq, Michel. *The Elementary Particles*. Translated by Frank Wynne. New York: Vintage, 2001.
  This extract will show you what kind of book this is: "The first night at Chris and Manu's left an extremely vivid impression on Bruno. Next to the dance floor were several rooms, bathed in a strange violet light. Beds were arranged close to each other. Everywhere, couples were having sex, stroking, and kissing. Most of the women were naked." This was the book that made conversations about swinging almost banal. In French, the description *houellebecquien* now applies to anything that suggests the sexualization of society.

- Millet, Catherine. *The Sexual Life of Catherine M.* Translated by Adriana Hunter. New York: Grove Press, 2003.
  To this day, Catherine Millet remains the woman who has spoken the most honestly and clearly about her taste for multiple partners. Now that the media circus has died down, her book deserves to be reread, for it will surely become a classic of erotica.

- Roché, Henri-Pierre. *Jules and Jim*. Translated by Patrick Evans. London: Marion Boyars, 1981.
  This is the novel that formed the basis for François Truffaut's classic film. It is the story of a love triangle, and it is much more romantic than erotic.

A THREE-PERSON PARTY

This account of a threesome is from Jacques Cellard's novel *Les petites marchandes de plaisir* (The Merchant-Girls of Pleasure). A prostitute, Lulu Bath, is telling her friend Pieu, the heroine of the novel, about a threesome in which she took part:

"We go up to the room reserved for parties of three and *tableaux vivants*, with its big bed. He puts two coins on the mantelpiece, fifteen francs. He lets himself be groomed, and then declares, a little sheepishly: 'I have a confession to make, my little angels. Never before have I made love to two women.'

"Irma, as she takes her shirt off, says, 'Don't tell me that you're frightened, Mr. Raoul.'

"'Frightened of you? Of course not. But I'm not familiar with the practice, and worry that I will seem a fool.'

"As I stretch out on the bed, I say, 'What an idea! You, seem foolish! Watch—I'll help you. Or would you rather make love to each of us in turn while pawing the other?'

"'No... No thank you.'

"I responded, 'But, my dear, you won't feel awkward giving us both pleasure, will you? I don't want to give away all our little secrets, Irma, but you know, when Mr. Raoul comes to see me, he usually takes a second helping.'

"'It's true, 'Mr. Raoul says. 'I had seconds the first time we met. We went at it twice on several other occasions, two or three times each month, sometimes beginning with a regular session, sometimes with an extraordinary one.'

"Says Irma: 'You have two sessions with her? So what difference does it make, Mr. Seconds, whether it's her and her or her and me?'

"'And I haven't told you the best part, Irma. Can I, dear Mr. Raoul? ... Well, he does it once here and once there, my dear. And he doesn't joke around. His is made of steel.'

"Irma leans toward him to see it for herself. I get her to climb onto the bed and I move away. And I suggest: 'My girl, show our friend your pussy. I would be shocked if he continued to dilly-dally after seeing it.'

"She mounts him and stands above his head, her legs wide open. Irma likes to let herself be seen by men. She's often told me that it excites her. ... Still uncomfortable in this new position, Mr. Raoul stops talking. In order to encourage him, I ask, 'Doesn't my friend have a pretty cooch? Oh, you can admire it. I'm not jealous. And if you look at it in the right way, it will grow wet, you know.'

"Then I went ahead and sat on that famous steel needle. Eh. It's only so-so. There are some men who get as hard as stone when there are two women, and some who go soft. He was between the two. But there's a remedy.

"'Oh, I'll bring your soldier back to life, Mr. Raoul! ... Part your lips, Irma, so that your button comes out nicely. I'm going to play his flute.'

"No sooner said than done. Mr. Raoul seizes Irma by her behind and now offers very flattering comments on the beauty of what he sees. My flute-playing yields the desired effect: [H]e becomes as hard as a young man. Irma begins to moan and asks, 'Can I jerk off, Lulu? I can't stand to be looked at so well any longer. Yes? Oh, I'm going to come, I'm going to come. Mr. Raoul, take...take it out!'"

IMAGES We also suggest you take a look at collections of old erotic images. Photographers have been taking erotic pictures since the dawn of photography, and even before then, plenty of cultures created sculptures and paintings depicting sex positions. Some will amaze you, either because of their beauty or their difficulty, and these enterprising artists of centuries past might even inspire you to try some new positions.

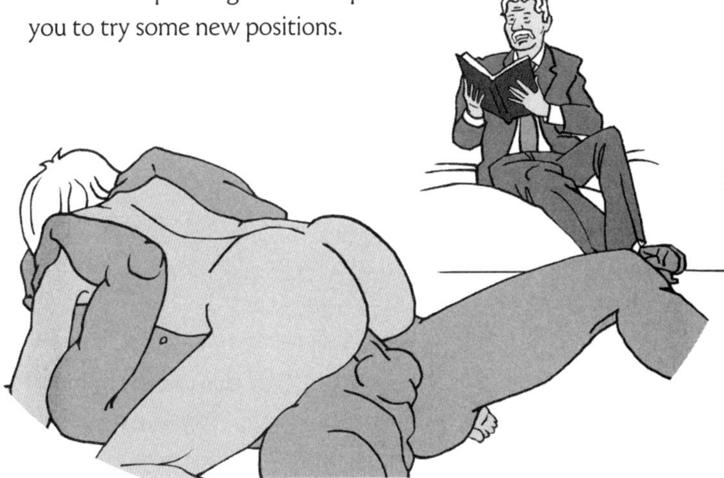

FIGURE 8.1. **A little exploration into the world of eroticism can make your sexual experiences that much more enjoyable.**

◎ **Films for Your Night Table** Even without counting porn, in which threesomes are standard issue, the *ménage à trois* has been a part of many films. Interestingly, it predominates in those from two eras. The first wave, from the sixties, tends to depict these living arrangements as sexual utopias, natural expressions of sexuality. The second wave, from this century, emphasizes the transgressive nature of the *ménage à trois*.

- *Blow-Up*. Directed by Michelangelo Antonioni, 1966. (With David Hemmings, Vanessa Redgrave, Peter Bowles, Sarah Miles, John Castle, Jane Birkin, Gillian Hills.)
  Blow-Up, about a fashion photographer's chance discovery of a murder, gave us the first opportunity to see Jane Birkin totally nude on-screen, in a threesome. It isn't the central theme of the movie, which is more concerned with voyeurism and photography, but the multiple partners in that sex scene caused a scandal when the film came out.

- *Douches froides* (Cold Showers). Directed by Antony Cordier, 2005. (With Johan Libéreau, Salomé Stévenin, Pierre Perier.)
  About young judo competitors in the midst of adolescent torments, *Cold Showers* features Salomé Stévenin as the beautiful Vanessa, who finds herself making love to her two friends, Clément and Mickael, on the rough floor of a judo dojo. "The first film with no errors in casting," said French magazine *Inrockuptibles*. "*Cold Showers* rethinks the dynamics behind threesomes and reveals the social mechanisms surrounding eroticism. Antony Cordier has the rare talent of being able to eroticize everything: class struggle, judo, crisis, shower gel."

- *The Dreamers*. Directed by Bernardo Bertolucci, 2003. (With Michael Pitt, Louis Garrel, Eva Green.)
  Paris, during the student strikes of May 1968. "The youths dream of a better world as they philosophize in cafés. The movement hardens and is violently repressed by police forces. It's against this backdrop that we meet Théo and his twin sister, Isabelle. French children of an English mother, they live in a wealthy bourgeois neighborhood near the Eiffel Tower. They meet Matthew, an American student who shares their passion for film, contemporary novels, the revolutionary spirit, thoughts about liberty, and sexuality." *The Dreamers* depicts a three-way relationship with a helping of possible incest between a twin brother (Louis Garrel) and sister (Eva Green).

- *Ken Park*. Directed by Larry Clark, 2003. (With Tiffany Limos, James Ransone, Stephen Jasso, James Bullard, Mike Apaletegui.)
  In Visalia, a small Californian town, a group of middle-class teenagers try to escape ennui through sex, violence, and perversion. A thought-provoking film, two scenes caused controversy: one involving a man masturbating and the final sequence, which shows a threesome—too short, but unsimulated—that remains to this day the most realistic and erotic depiction of multiple partners.

ON TELEVISION

- *Sex and the City*, "Three's a Crowd" (Season 1, episode 8)
  It was inevitable that the four single New York ladies of *Sex and the City* would wonder about threesomes. Carrie discovers that Mr. Big used to be married and, moreover, that he and his ex-wife took part in a threesome. Charlotte's

boyfriend wants to invite another woman into their bed. As to Samantha, she finds herself in the midst of a married couple. Our friends are disturbed, but as usual, Samantha winds up taking a view that combines philosophical attitudes and delicacy.

Safer Sex Some information on safer sex practices to keep in mind with multiple-partner sex can be found at the following websites and in Tristan Taormino's book *Opening Up*.

The Body: http://www.thebody.com

The Centers for Disease Control (CDC), National Prevention Information Network: http://www.cdcnpin.org/scripts/hiv/index.asp

Conclusion What happens afterward?

My little book has been written entirely in the hedonistic vein. I've focused on the pleasurable side of things and have let moral critics fall by the wayside. But remember, there are consequences to having sex with multiple partners, and you need to consider them carefully. One of the most significant is simply that you'll develop a taste for it. Wanting to have sex only in these situations may seriously complicate your love life. That's where swingers clubs come in. There, no one will be surprised by your behavior, even if society at large thinks it is beyond the pale. No one will judge you, and that's the most important part.

Going to swingers clubs isn't quite as nice as going to someone's house, but at least you're guaranteed anonymity. After all, how can you be sure that one of the three men you took home one night won't tell his friends about your feats and ruin your reputation in the process? So be careful, especially if you find yourself in the company of strangers. As one of our interlocutors said, "The downside of having sex with two other people is the same as that of having sex with one person—only worse."

I also want to warn you once more about STIs. The more people you have in bed and the more often you have them, the greater your risk. So use a rubber and take care.

Once you've taken these precautions, you can go out with one goal: to have sex with a bunch of people. And remember, no matter how many people you have in bed, it is still sex.

Bibliography

Alter, Anna, and Perrine Cherchève. *Super positions* (Super Positions). Paris: Hachette Littérature, 2003.

Anonymous. *Les Pucelages conquis: ou, Scènes libres de ce qui se passait dans les couvents d'Italie au moment de leur suppression, en 1808* (Conquered Virginity, or, Scenes of What Occurred in Italian Convents at the Moment of Their Suppression in 1808). Paris: Chez les marchands de nouveautès, 1850(?).

Anonymous. *The School for Girls*. No translation credit. New York: Olympia Press, 2005. Originally published as *L'Ecole des Biche*.

Argens, Marquis de. *Therese the Philosopher*. No translation credit. New York: Olympia Press, 2007. Originally published as *Thérèse Philosophe*.

Arsan, Emmanuelle. *Emmanuelle*. Paris: La Musardine, 1999.

Barbe, Hélène. *Osez… l'échangisme* (Dare… to Try Swinging). Paris: La Musardine, 2004

Bennett, Jessica. "Only You. And You. And You." *Newsweek*, 2009. http://www.newsweek.com/id/209164 (accessed 21 April 2010).

Biermann, Michael. *Les trentes jours de Marseille* (Thirty Days of Marseille). Paris: Le Cercle, 2001.

Bouyxou, Jean-Pierre. *Fascination: Le Musée secret de l'erotisme* (Fascination: The Secret Eroticism Museum) No. 5, 1979.

Cellard, Jacques. *Les petites marchandes de plaisir* (The Merchant-Girls of Pleasure). Paris: Éditions Balland, 1990.

Chorier, Nicolas. *The School of Women* (also published in English as *Dialogues of Luisa Sigea* and in French as *L'Academie des dames).* 1682.

Dannam, Marc, and Axterdam. *Dare... to Try Kama Sutra.* Alameda, CA: Hunter House, 2009.

de Nerciat, Andréa. *Félicia, ou mes fredaines* (Félicia, or My Mischief), 1772.

Dictionnaire de l'amour, de l'érotisme, et de la sexualité (Dictionary of Love, Erotica, and Sexuality). Paris: Editions Galea, 1980.

Duca, Lo. *Nouveau dictionnaire de sexologie* (The New Dictionary of Sexology). Paris: Éditions L'Or du temps, 1967.

Esparbec. *Les Main baladeuses* (Wandering Hands). Paris: La Musardine, 2004.

Étienne, Charles Guillaume. *Notre-Dame de Lesbos.* Paris: Editions Curio, 1929.

Ferroul, Yves. La sexualité féminine (Female Sexuality). Paris: Ellipses Marketing, 2002.

Fur, Gala. *Osez... tout savoir sur le SM* (Dare... to Learn Everything about S&M). Paris: La Musardine, 2004.

Iacub, Marcela. *Le Crime était presque sexuel* (The Crime Was Almost Sexual). Paris: Éditions Epel, 2002.

________. *Qu'avez-vous fait de la libération sexuelle?* (What Have You Done With Sexual Liberation?) Paris: Flammarion, 2002.

Lefort, Gérard. Article in French magazine *Libération* (1 August 2005).

Lemonier, Marc. *Mangeuses d'hommes* (The Man-Eating Women). Paris: La Musardine, in press.

"Le Sexe en Questions," (Sex in Questions) *20 Ans* (20 Years Old) 225, (June 2005).

Linux, Elsa. *Le journal d'Elsa Linux* (Elsa Linux's Diary). Paris: La Musardine, 2005.

Louÿs, Pierre. *Histoire du roi Gonzalve et des douze princesses.* Paris: La Musardine, 1996.

Love, Brenda. *Encyclopedia of Unusual Sex Practices.* New York: Barricade Books, 1994.

Morisset, Josée-Gabrielle. Article in Canadian lesbian magazine *Corps et Âme* (Body and Soul), April 2003.

Martin Van Maële. *Alors tu y as été souvent au bordel?* (So, you've been often to the brothel?) In *La Grande danse macabre des vifs* (The Grand Macabre Dance of the Dead). Charles Carrington, 1905.

Millet, Catherine. *The Sexual Life of Catherine M.* Translated by Adriana Hunter. New York: Grove Press, 2003. Originally published as *La vie sexuelle de Catherine M.* (Paris: Éditions du Seuil, 2001).

Money, John. *Love and Love Sickness*. Baltimore, MD: The Johns Hopkins University Press, 1980.

Mossuz-Lavau, Janine. *La Vie sexuelle en France* (Sexual Life in France). Paris: La Martinière, 2002.

Musset, Alfred de. *Gamiani, or Two Nights of Excess*. New York: Olympia Press, 2007.

Ovidie. *Osez… tourner votre film X* (Dare… to Make an X-Rated Film). Paris: La Musardine, 2005.

Rambal, Julia. "Ce que révèlent nos fantasmes" (What Our Fantasies Tell Us). *Bien dans ma vie* (Feeling Good in Life), August 2005.

Rozen, Anna. *Plaisir d'offrir, joie de reçevoir* (The Pleasure of Giving, the Joy of Receiving). Paris: Le Dilettante, 1999.

Taormino, Tristan. *Opening Up: A Guide to Creating and Sustaining Open Relationships.* Berkeley, CA: Cleis Press, 2008.

Vian, Boris. *Écrits pornographiques (1947–1958)* (Pornographic Writings). Paris: C Bourgois, 1980.

Welzer-Lang, Daniel. *La planète échangiste: Les sexualités collectives en France* (Swingers Planet: Group Sexuality in France). Paris: Éditions Payot, 2005.